ATTENTION

DEFICIT

DISORDER

by Glenn Hunsucker, M. A.

Printed in the United States of America

Forresst Publishing is a division of Glenn Hunsucker, Professional Corporation. P. O. Box 7046, Abilene, Texas 79608

ISBN 09619650-0-2

First Printing, 1988

Second Printing, 1988

ACKNOWLEDGEMENTS

I would like to thank everyone with whom I have had contact in compiling this book. There are too many to mention by name but I would like to thank them all.

A special thanks to Betty Anderson and her family, Troy and Matt, for the long hours she has put in.

Thanks to all of the youngsters and families whom I've treated. This book would not have been possible without you.

DEDICATION

I would like to dedicate this book to the thousands of individuals who have had an Attention Deficit Disorder (ADD) but were never treated. Their lives may have been spared untold pain and suffering. In some instances, their lives may have been spared if they had received the proper treatment.

Ironically, if it had not been for the pain and suffering of these overlooked individuals, I would not have had the intestinal fortitude to put forth the effort to compile the information in this book. If this book helps one person, the effort was worth it.

CONTENTS

I. PURPOSE AND SCOPE OF THIS BOOK   1

II. DESCRIPTION OF ADD   7

III. CAUSES OF ADD   15
     Heredity
     Physiological
     Psychosocial

IV. PROBLEM AREAS   21
     Physical
     Academic
     Behavior
     Emotional
     Social

V. FAMILY DYNAMICS   33
     Psychiatric Problems
     Siblings
     Parents

VI. ADD FROM BIRTH TO ADULTHOOD   49
     Infancy
     Pre-school Years
     Entering School
     Adolescence
     Adulthood

VII. EVALUATION   61
     Parent Questionnaire
     Teacher Questionnaire
     Medical/Social History of Child
     Medical/Social History of Parents
     Observational Methods
     Other Techniques

VIII. TREATMENT   81
       Medication
       Behavioral Management
       Other Treatment Methods

  IX. IMPROVEMENTS SEEN AFTER MEDICATION   99
       Academic/Learning
       Behavior
       Emotional

   X. DEALING WITH OTHER AGENCIES   103
       School Systems
       Department of Human Services
       Juvenile Probation Department
       Adoption Agencies
       Children's Homes

  XI. REASONS ADD MAY BE OVERLOOKED   121

 XII. QUESTIONS AND ANSWERS   125

XIII. CASE REPORTS   143

       FINAL COMMENT

       REFERENCES

CHAPTER I

PURPOSE AND SCOPE OF THIS BOOK

The reason that I included this part of the book as a chapter instead of a foreword, is because I feel it is important for you to understand some of the reasoning involved in writing the book. Also, I discovered that most people skip the foreword and go directly to Chapter I anyway.

I would like to briefly state how I became involved with this disorder. When I finished graduate school, I went directly into private practice. I worked for a psychologist who had two other associates. Because I was new in the field, I was given the youngsters who were referred to the office. Most of these children were having either behavioral or academic problems. I also received referrals from Juvenile Probation Departments. These youngsters were obvious behavior problems.

Since I had a Master's Degree in Psychology, I felt confident that I was armed with sufficient knowledge to "cure" these children and their families. I was familiar with behavioral modification techniques which I was ready to pass on to the parents in order to help them "cure" their children. If this didn't work, I was also armed with counseling techniques that I was sure would help either the children or parents. I was also under the impression that if a child was having any kind of problem, it was probably the parents' fault. After a few months of working under these assumptions, I discovered that something was definitely wrong with my theory.

I found that the behavioral management techniques that I suggested the parents use, had already been tried. The parents were a lot smarter than I thought. My decision at that point was to try and counsel the parents. Strangely enough, the parents stayed in counseling, but the child's behavior did not change. I began searching and grasping at straws because I was not having the success I expected. I began to doubt my competence. I also began to doubt the usefulness of my college education. After a year or so, I started to notice some similarities among the children. Some had been on medication for a short time and most had some kind of learning problems. This inspired my interest in learning disabilities and eventually Attention Deficit Disorder (ADD). I am amazed to this day, that many of my colleagues have an incomplete knowledge of this disorder. Even in graduate school, ADD was hardly mentioned.

Needless to say, this is when I became involved in the diagnosis and treatment of these children. I was beginning to feel that I had found a breakthrough until I encountered a number of unforseen problems with other agencies when trying to treat these children. These problems are numerous and will be mentioned throughout the book.

I would now like to comment on the fact that I am not a medical doctor, yet I am writing

about a disorder that seems to be in the domain
of the medical community.

I have discovered that the majority of children
with ADD are referred to someone like myself
due to the presence of other problems. They are
not referred to see if they have ADD. Therefore,
I see it as crucial for therapists to fully understand
ADD.

Both physicians and therapists have their
expertise. Unfortunately, in order to diagnose
and treat ADD properly, it requires a working
knowledge of both areas. Finding a person with
this unique combination of skills is rare.

This is why I'm writing this book. Parents
as well as professionals should be able to see
how ADD needs to be treated by both physiological
and psychological methods. It will take the co-
ordinated effort of professionals to properly diagnose and treat these children.

I am going to make some statements in this
chapter that may sound ridiculous and melodra-
matic. These statements are the result of my
experiences in dealing with Attention Deficit
Disorder (A.D.D.)

I have collected numerous research articles
on A.D.D. and they are listed in the references.
I am writing this book for the lay person while
including scientifically sound research material
to appeal to the professional. However, I can
assure you that the professional who thrives on
technical terminology will cringe at some of my
examples and analogies.

I try to separate what is my theory with what is supported by research. However, much of my theory is based on the research of others as well as empirical evidence. I will now stick out my neck and make the following statements.

If every person who has A.D.D. were treated at an early age, I feel there would be a substantial reduction in the following areas:

1. Reduction in crime rate (adult & juvenile).
2. Reduction in school drop out rate.
3. Reduction in alochol & other drug abuse.

As you read the book, I believe you will understand the rationale behind these statements. I feel that a lot of other areas would be affected also. However, these three areas would be most obviously affected.

There has been a great deal of research on ADD in the past twenty years. The researchers have made important discoveries regarding the areas I have previously mentioned. I feel that one of the reasons that no one has stated what I am stating, is due to fear of criticism. As you can see, I have made some rather bold statements. I feel that most people would look at these and conclude that I think I have the answer to the world's problems. It sounds like a panacea. I agree, it does sound rather dramatic that these areas could be improved upon by properly treating one Disorder (ADD). However, after reading the research and seeing the dramatic changes in my clients, I feel my claims are warranted.

The only thing I am doing differently than the scientific community, is making <u>definite</u> statements. Researchers disguise their conclusions in such qualifying terms that it becomes difficult to determine exactly what they are saying. They appear to be writing for the benefit of other researchers. They try to avoid making statements that sound too definitive. They use qualifying words so often that their main point is lost. In actuality, their research suggests that my assertions are correct. I am convinced that there are hundreds of thousands of individuals in the United States who have suffered needlessly. If this book helps one individual diagnose him or herself and seek treatment, then my brash statements are worth it. If it helps one parent diagnose their child and seek treatment, then my brash statements are worth it.

The field of psychology and counseling has gained a much wider acceptance in the past twenty years. There are more mental health professionals than in the history of the United States. Churches now provide counseling and almost every college has a counseling service for the public. There are more awareness campaigns than there has ever been. Yet, can anyone point to any of the areas that I mentioned previously and say that there has been a significant improvement? Is the crime rate going down? Are fewer students dropping out of school? Has alcohol and other drug abuse decreased? Has juvenile crime decreased? The answer is no! My contention is that something is wrong with the way these problems have been handled. I feel that one thing that has been handled wrong is the diagnosis of ADD. This is supported by case studies done by others and which are presented in this book. I am not saying that everyone who has had problems in the areas mentioned, had ADD. I am saying that if one common thread could be found among the individuals in these groups, I feel that ADD would be far ahead of any other diagnostic category. Consequently, a proper treatment of everyone with this disorder could have a significant impact on these areas.

Again, I know this sounds rather bold to suggest that one disorder can affect so many different areas. At times, I question whether or not I am obsessed with this disorder and can't see anything else. But, when I see the dramatic results in the children I have treated, knowing that the course of their lives has probably been changed, I am almost certain I am correct.

Believe me, I am not the only person who feels that ADD is overlooked. I will say that I am probably one of the few who is willing to stick out his neck and make such broad sweeping statements. I am also willing to state that millions of our tax dollars are being wasted every year because ADD is being overlooked. Juvenile probation departments, the departments of Human Services, and public school systems are the major culprits. They spend money for treatment methods that are inappropriate for these youngsters. In essence, they are responsible for most of our youth being "mistreated." This will be mentioned in a little more detail within the book.

I repeat certain facts throughout the book. This is because I see these particular facts as extremely important and I want the reader to remember them. Therefore, please bear with the redundant statements.

CHAPTER II

DESCRIPTION OF ADD

Before I explain the symptoms of this disorder, I must first give you some background information.

Although many of you may not be familiar with the term Attention Deficit Disorder (ADD), you are probably familiar with the term hyperactivity. Hyperactivity used to be the term used for children who are now diagnosed as ADD. Other terms that were used before hyperactivity were minimal brain damage, hyperkinesis, and the broad label of learning disabled. You may wonder why the name was changed to ADD. It may seem that the name was changed in order to be more stylish. Actually, the reason for the change is logical, and is beneficial to the many children who may otherwise be overlooked when other terms are used.

Through research, it was discovered there were a number of children who exhibited the same problems that hyperactive children exhibited but, they were not overly active. In other words, they had short attention spans, had difficulty concentrating, and difficulty with school work, but they did not bounce off the wall. Therefore, the diagnostic category of hyperactivity did not fit these children. These children were overlooked. Consequently it was discovered that the major problem with these children, including the hyperactive children, was their attention. Hence, the name Attention Deficit Disorder was used to include both the hyperactive and non-hyperactive children.

Under this broad category of Attention Deficit Disorder, three levels were identified. ADD with hyperactivity, ADD without hyperactivity, and ADD residual type. (This has recently been changed.)

ADD with hyperactivity is the equivalent of the often used diagnosis Hyperactivity.

ADD without hyperactivity was used to include the children who had attentional problems, but were not necessarily overactive.

ADD residual type includes persons who may have had ADD as a child and must now deal with the emotional or psychological problems that have resulted from having this disorder without having been treated.

As previously mentioned, the major difficulty of children with ADD is attentional. They have difficulty maintaining attention in the classroom as well as at home. They are impulsive and have difficulty sticking with tasks for long periods of time. They are disorganized and do not complete their work at school or at home. Their school work is usually sloppy and inaccurate. These children may be seen as not listening to what they have been told. They sometimes seem to lack common sense and overlook the obvious.

These children usually have more problems in a group situation than when they are one on one. The reason that group situations seem to be difficult for these children is because they are easily distracted both visually and auditorily. Parents may have a difficult time getting the child to obey or follow through on directives. The parent may discover that these children have trouble sticking to one play activity for any period of time. These children are prone to have temper outbursts and unpredictable behaviors. Parents may sometimes worry that these children have no conscience. They may have difficulty keeping friends because they usually play rougher than the average child. The more overly active children may sometimes appear to have never ending energy. It is sometimes hard to get them to take a nap, and they appear to need less sleep than most children.

At this point I must state that all children exhibit the traits previously mentioned. However, the difference between the average child and an ADD child is one of degree.

What I am describing is behavior that exceeds that of the average child. You may wonder exactly what does the average child do. As this book continues, the differences will become more obvious. A general rule of thumb is that the behavior of ADD children is not goal directed. This means that their activity is usually not organized toward a predictable end result. Because their attention jumps from one area to another, they usually do not complete a task.

To confuse you more, I will state that this disorder is not exactly the same in every child. For example, a child may do well at school and poorly at home or vice versa. One child may have learning problems to a severe degree, while another

child may not exhibit such obvious learning problems. One child may exhibit these problems
at the age of three or four years, while another
child may not exhibit school difficulties until
the seventh or eighth grade.

Because the symptoms differ from child to
child, diagnosing ADD is sometimes difficult.

ADD is a common disorder among children.
This is an important piece of information. I am
not writing about a disorder that occurs less often
than other problems. Research shows that between
three to five percent of children have this disorder.
Some estimates go as high as ten percent. Although
this does not sound like a large number, let me
give you a comparison of disorders with which
you are more familiar. For example, mentally
retarded individuals (adults and children) make
up one percent of the total population. Remember,
we are including adults in this one percent. That
means, that if we were to remove the adults
from this figure and include only children, the
percentage of mentally retarded would be well
below one percent. As previously stated, ADD
is estimated to be three to ten percent of the
population of children. Adults are not included
in this number.

Consequently the number of children with
ADD is from six to twenty times that of the
children with mental retardation.

Why is it then, there are special programs
for the mentally retarded yet ADD, a more common problem is overlooked? One obvious answer
is that a person who is mentally retarded is more
easily identified than a child with ADD. Also,
children who are mentally retarded exhibit obvious

intellectual deficits that can be readily identified through achievement and I.Q. tests. This is not the case with ADD.

Although these children have attentional problems and are impulsive, they are not necessarily less intelligent. In fact, many have an extremely high level of intelligence and are rather creative. These children appear to do poorly in the classroom, not because of a lack of intelligence, but because of their short term memory, short attention span, and distractibility. This makes it hard for them to concentrate on and complete tasks.

On individually administered I.Q. tests, they perform well and usually do not qualify for special educational placement. Because the child does not qualify for special educational placement, they are often required to remain in regular classes. Although they may be struggling with certain courses, or perhaps failing, the school system may not allow them special education because the reasons for their failure are not readily identified. Many teachers or counselors may feel that the child is merely lazy or oppositional.

Many times it is suspected that these children have auditory processing problems because they don't seem to hear directives. However, it is usually their short attention span and not an auditory problem that accounts for this "hearing" problem. It is probably a good idea to send the child for hearing tests, or other auditory tests to rule out this explanation.

Many of these children have been found to have poor speech development. Again, not all children, just some. These children, especially

the ones with hyperactivity, are said to have
little appreciation for the social, ethical, moral,
or even legal consequences of their behavior.
Right and wrong do not seem to govern their
actions. They do not seem to respect other people's
feelings or property.

ADD children without hyperactivity may
be totally opposite.....they may be guilt-ridden,
down on themselves, or give their toys away.
They will not try to push themselves into situations
with other people and many times they may be
seen as a nerd, shy, or withdrawn. Therefore,
it is not easy to pinpoint a child with ADD just
based on their social functioning. As was mentioned
earlier, one child may manifest symptoms of
the disorder in one manner while another may
manifest symptoms in an opposite manner.

This disorder is ten times more common in
boys than in girls. It also appears to be more
common among the 1st born. The disorder is also
hereditary. This means that there is likely to
be a history of academic or behavior problems
in the family. Drug usage (alcohol) is also common
in the family history. Research shows that ADD
may predispose a person to becoming an alcoholic
or drug abuser. Children with ADD are likely
to have academic problems and/or social problems.
In other words, they may have trouble functioning
in a group of peers. However, the confusing thing
about the disorder is that they may do well in
one area but poorly in another.

Some of these children may exhibit a low
tolerance for frustration and have mood swings.
They sometimes develop low self-esteem and
school drop out rates among youngsters with ADD
is very high. Research also indicates that teenagers

who have ADD are more likely to become involved in juvenile crime.

The disorder sometimes may disappear by puberty. Other times some symptoms, such as excessive over activity, may disappear but attentional problems remain. Unfortunately, it is not uncommon for all of the symptoms to continue throughout adult life.

The following is a list of symptoms common to ADD children with hyperactivity.

1. They have trouble concentrating on things for a long period of time.
2. They become easily distracted (visually/auditorily).
3. They have trouble following directions.
4. They do not finish what they start.
5. They act before they think.
6. They need more supervision than other children.
7. They are usually disruptive in class.
8. They do not like to wait their turn in games.
9. They go from one activity to another and have trouble sticking to one play activity.
10. Signs of the disorder are evident before age 7.
11. Loses things (i.e., school work, books, etc.)
12. Answers questions before they are completed.
13. Squirms or fidgets (teenagers may feel restless.)
14. Engages in risk taking behavior.
15. Intrudes on conversations.
16. Trouble following through on directions.
17. May talk excessively.
18. Overall disorganization or extremely organized.

ADD children without hyperactivity exhibit the following symptoms.

1. They have trouble concentrating on things for a long period of time.
2. Easily distracted.
3. They have trouble following directions.
4. They do not finish what they start (although they may try harder than those who are hyperactive.)
5. They lose things (i.e., school work, books, etc.)
6. Overall disorganization or overly organized.
7. Seem to be depressed and daydream a great deal.
8. May be meek and not speak out in defense of themselves as their hyperactive counterparts might.

CHAPTER III

CAUSES OF ADD

Attention Deficit Disorder, with or without hyperactivity, is a neurological problem. It does not occur in the muscles, arms, or legs. It occurs in the brain. I include this section in the book in order to answer some questions some people may have. I personally feel that the causes of ADD are not as important as the treatment. It is known that this disorder is a chemical imbalance and is hereditary. It has also been shown that medication is the only treatment that has been effective. I will now cover some areas that have been highly publicized in recent years as the causes of ADD.

HEREDITY

Research indicates that the families of ADD children show a history of alcoholism, illegal behavior, and depression. The siblings of ADD children are more likely to have similar problems. Studies have been done on twins that point to the conclusion that the disorder is obtained genetically.

Unfortunately, when the aforementioned traits of the family members are listed (i.e., alcoholism, depression), most people conclude that this type of environment is probably responsible for the child having ADD. This may make sense until you remember that this is a <u>neurological</u> problem. If a child exhibits problems in this environment but then is changed to another environment where his problems disappear, the child probably didn't have ADD in the first place.

Heredity explains where a child obtains ADD but does not explain how it occurred in the first individual who passed it on down the line. This is still a mystery.

PHYSIOLOGICAL FACTORS

This area seems to be the most studied by professionals. Nutritionists swear that food additives and refined sugars have a lot to do with this disorder. They are usually referring to hyperactive children. It is obvious that sugar does create agitation among children with this disorder. It is questionable whether or not this is the <u>cause</u> of the disorder. Reducing a child's intake of sugar will not automatically cure ADD. Remember, the only treatment that has been found to be effective is medication.

Lead poisoning has also been questioned as a problem causing ADD. There has not been enough scientific evidence to suggest that this is the case. There has been speculation for years that flourescent lighting causes children to be more hyperactive. This may be the case, but children with ADD perform just as poorly in settings that do not include flourescent lighting. Smoking and drinking during pregnancy has also been thought to be a cause of this disorder. Again, it may have a negative impact on the child, but it has not been found to be the primary cause of ADD.

Some researchers believe that the major difficulty in the brain is with the neurotransmitters. I am not a scientist or a medical doctor, but I will try to relate to you in terms that I understand, what this means. The brain has millions of neurons. In between these neurons is a chemical called a neurotransmitter. This relays messages of pain, memory, and other human actions. Scientists feel that the major problem is this chemical between the neurons. Hence, a chemical imbalance. The only way that the chemical can be balanced is by the introduction of another chemical. This means that medication must be used. Research has become so exact that they feel they have located the part of the brain that is the major problem. This appears to be the pre-frontal cortex. They know that the pre-frontal cortex plays a role in the planning and regulating of complex human behavior. It allows humans to anticipate and prepare for future events. Researchers have noted that people that have had injuries to the pre-frontal cortex have problems similar to that of ADD children. They are inattentive, distractible, impulsive, and unable to follow rules. Although it cannot be stated as a matter of fact that the problem is with the neurotransmitter, evidence does point to this being the primary problem.

PSYCHOSOCIAL FACTORS

Many people do not feel that this is a physiological problem at all. They think that the child is disruptive and impulsive because the parents have not done a good job in raising their child. This view is the primary reason many kids are overlooked as having ADD.

Teachers, pediatricians, therapists, etc., assume that there is some psychological reason that the child is not doing well in school or is a behavior problem.

This is especially true if the child in question is a teenager and has been overlooked for years. Professionals assume that if ADD was the problem it would have been discovered years ago. Therefore, the explanation for the child's behavior or poor academic performance must lie with their emotional environment. In other words, the parents.

If there happens to be some personal problems within the family, this only reinforces the view that the parents are the problem. Research indicates that there are likely to be more problems within families of ADD children. But, these problems were not the cause of the child inheriting a physiological problem.

Another problem that arises is if the child is adopted and starts having problems. The assumption is that they are suffering from a sense of separation from their natural parents. Although this may occur, I have found that this is rarely the case. The major reason these children are having problems is related to the characteristics of ADD.

In essence, I feel that as a society, we have learned to "psychologize" too much. We can give an explanation for everything that a person does. These explanations may sound logical and realistic. However, this doesn't mean that they are correct. For example, there is not a family in the United States that doesn't have some kind of problem areas. In other words, I could go into anyone's household and point out something that needs to be changed because of the negative "psychological" impact that this will have upon the child. My reasoning may sound logical but not necessarily be correct. This is especially true of families with ADD children. Since research shows that these families may be more disorganized than others, they are prime targets for those professionals who enjoy "psychologizing."

My major point is this: If a child has ADD, there is absolutely no way that this can be caused by a psychological or social event. The problems of ADD children can be influenced by psychological and social factors as any other child can be influenced. However, ADD is a hereditary physiological problem that can only successfully be treated through the use of medication. Removing psychological or social problems from the child's life will not "cure" the disorder. If it does, they never had ADD in the first place.

CHAPTER IV

PROBLEM AREAS

There seem to be several areas in which children have problems. The different areas will be listed below:

1. Physical
2. Academic
3. Behavioral
4. Emotional
5. Social

PHYSICAL PROBLEMS

A great deal of research has been done on physical problems of ADD children. Because hyperactivity was identified years ago, most of the research has been done on these children. ADD is thought to be neurological, therefore much physical research has been done. Research does show there may be more physical immaturity in these children than in non-ADD children. They have found, especially among hyperactive children, that they are smaller and thinner than others their age. Some of the research has shown that even their bone structure is immature. That is, they grow slower and are behind in development in comparison to other children. Neurological examinations indicate slight hints of a problem, but this is not a conclusive piece of evidence that would allow a researcher to state that there only are identifiable neurological problems. This does suggest neurological immaturity.

Many of these children may be uncoordinated. ADD children for the most part, need less sleep than other children, especially the hyperactive ones. I have seen numerous ADD children who are ambidextrous. Again, I am not a brain specialist, but this does suggest that they have not developed hemispheric dominance as quickly as other children.

There have been reports from parents that they must take extreme measures to keep them in control. This was true even as an infant. Many times the parents may find the child in the bathroom going through the medicine cabinet while everyone else is still asleep.

ADD children have been known to have more physical ailments than other children. They seem to have more colds, upper respiratory problems, allergies, and ear infections. Many of these children are not good in the athletic arena. However, some are very good athletes, and are more durable than others. Research indicates that these children receive more broken bones and bruises than other children. I feel that this is probably due to the fact that they have a high tolerance for pain. Consequently they do not try to avoid obstacles or situations that other children avoid. They appear to be fearless or not able to recognize dangerous situations. Because of their risk taking attitude, they will approach any situation without fear.

I have found that many of these children
are bed wetters. Why this is the case I tend to
lean toward an explanation that relates to their
high tolerance for pain. Many times, the reason
a child wets the bed is because he is unable to
feel the pressure of the bladder expanding. When
the bladder expands, it causes pain and consequently causes the child to wake up and use the
restroom. If they have a high tolerance for pain,
it is unlikely that they will be alerted to the
need. Again this is my opinion regarding the reasons
for bedwetting, but I have seen no studies which
support my theory.

ACADEMIC PROBLEMS

At this point I must distinguish between ADD
children with hyperactivity and ADD children
without hyperactivity. ADD children with hyperactivity are usually disruptive and noncompliant
in the classroom. They are out of their seat more
often than other children. They disrupt others
and they cannot stay at a task for long periods
of time.

ADD children without hyperactivity may
be compliant and sit, staring out the window,
or just lean back as if they are not going to attempt their work. They may just sit there and
look frustrated. These children may not be as
troublesome to teachers as are their hyperactive
counterparts. They may have the same basic problems (i.e., trouble concentrating, easily distracted)
but they are not overly active. Unfortunately,
these children may not come to the attention
of the teacher as quickly as the disruptive child.
Consequently, the disruptive child may receive
help by being referred for testing, or a parent-

teacher conference may result in the parent seeking outside help. The more complacent ADD child may continue to be overlooked for years. In fact, the teacher may comment on what a tremendous child the parents have. If the teacher likes the child, there is a chance that the child will be granted higher grades than they deserve. The teacher probably feels they are doing the child a favor. Unfortunately, they are doing the child a disservice. I have seen many ADD children who did not come to my attention until they were in the 7th, 8th, or 9th grades. This was due to the fact that they had the kind of personality that most teachers enjoyed. Apparently, this influenced the manner in which the teacher graded them. They were passed, but their problems eventually caught up with them in the later years.

The explanation for a child who does behave, but makes poor grades, is many times seen as evidence of an emotional problem. When this conclusion is made, the parents are seen as the culprits. They may be seen as the cause of the child's problems.

When an ADD child reaches middle school (6th - 8th) their problems with concentration, organization, and distractibility may become more evident, even if they have been overlooked in previous years. Research shows that a large number of ADD children have learning problems or learning disabilities. They also have poor handwriting. These problems usually do not disappear as the child gets older. They may become masked. In other words, other problems may arise that direct attention away from the ADD. For example, after years of being frustrated and disappointed, an ADD child may gravitate toward negative behavior.

No one may ever suspect that ADD is the problem now. They are inclined to look at the child's behavior and then look for an environmental explanation (i.e., the parents.)

Problems which arise may include their not turning in their homework. They may have completed it and complain that it was turned in. Because of their short attention span, they may have forgotten to give it to the teachers. I have had parents tell me that, at the end of the school year, dozens of completed papers were found at the bottom of their child's locker. These papers were never turned in. Why does this happen? I have discovered that when an ADD child begins changing classes every hour, their lack of organizational skills begin to show. Consider that the child must now go to his locker every hour and get the books he needs as well as the homework for that class. At the end of the day the child must remember in which classes he has homework and get the appropriate book. By the end of the day, he may have forgotten. If he does remember, he may forget to get it out of his locker the next day when the time comes for that particular class.

Teachers sometimes complain that the child takes too much time to complete work. Other teachers complain that the child does it too quickly. This may sound contradictory, but children with ADD may have the same problems, but deal with them in different ways. One child may be so afraid of making a mistake that they go over their work again and again. Others may be so impulsive that they overlook details and hence, complete their work before everyone else. It is difficult for people to understand that these children may have the same problem.

Parents report that working with these children at home presents problems. They report that they become more frustrated than the child. An idea or concept may have to be stated several times before it is absorbed. After several minutes, the child may have already forgotten the concept. Parents report that after something is drilled into the child, they may never forget it, or the child takes it to extremes. It is as if the child takes things literally and is not able to generalize. Many parents consider this a lack of common sense. This is why school becomes more difficult for these children. The concepts with which they must work become more complicated in the higher grades.

Parents also complain that these children become frustrated when doing homework and may throw temper tantrums. They may have to spend an inordinate amount of time on their school work in order to make average grades. This will take its toll on the child after a number of years. As a matter of fact, I have noticed that these children's grades become progressively worse toward the middle and end of the school year. Sometimes, their grades may fluctuate from one grading period to another. I interpret this as their way of coping with the build-up of frustration. They sort of take a rest period after a period of intense concentration and effort. As their tolerance wears thin, their performance suffers.

BEHAVIORAL PROBLEMS

Impulsiveness and aggressive actions are some of the more commonly noted problems. ADD children with hyperactivity are usually more vocal and noisy in the classroom. They are sometimes disruptive both in class and at home. These children seem to have high risk taking behavior. That is, they will take chances that other children will not. Consequently, these children end up having more accidents, bumps and bruises, scrapes, and broken bones than other kids their age. These children do not seem to be able to appreciate the long or short term consequences of their behavior. They are after the thrill of doing something just out of curiosity. These children end up being frustrating to the parents who must supervise them constantly in order to prevent accidents. Many of these children, because they have an above average curiosity, end up taking toys apart just to see how they work. They do not always put them back together. Summertime is very difficult for parents because of the idle time these children have.

Contrary to the popular belief that positive reinforcement is a big motivating factor for children, the opposite is true for ADD children with hyperactivity. They respond better to negative feedback. In other words, you almost have to have a temper tantrum to get the child's attention and get them to respond to your request. I have discovered that many of the children with whom I have dealt, appear to have an abnormal threshold of pain. To explain further, many of these children have a high tolerance for pain. Therefore, spankings do not work. What would hurt children with normal pain thresholds, will not hurt these children. Consequently, they are not deterred by threats of physical punishment. After a spanking, they are likely to just turn around and say, "are you finished?", and then walk away and repeat the previous behavior. This becomes frustrating to parents and sometimes leads them to even more harsh punishment. These children have to be reminded to complete their chores more often than other children and are punished more often for non-compliance.

Because they have difficulty controlling their behavior and evaluating the consequences of their acts, they are prone to repeat this behavior in the future. This can have dramatic consequences for this person's life. The misbehaviors of a 6-year old are much different from the misbehaviors of a 16-year old.

Some ADD children may resort to being the class clown. I feel that this may occur due to their inability to achieve academically, so they try to achieve socially by performing humorous antics. It appears to be more socially acceptable to be considered a person who doesn't perform well in school because of their desire to be the center of attention rather than a person who has a learning problem.

EMOTIONAL PROBLEMS

The emotional aspects of children with ADD have been the least studied. Consequently, this has been my major focus over the past few years. Most professionals seem to under-estimate the emotional impact on someone going untreated over a number of years. The school system, which comes in contact with ADD children, usually focus more on the academics and not emotions. They become concerned when the child exhibits a behavior or academic problem.

The child who drops between the cracks is the ADD child without hyperactivity. They may be passing, yet the amount of time that they must spend studying is excessive. The frustration that this child feels cannot be measured by any test. For example, a child who has had ADD up until the sixth grade, and has been passing, has experienced six years of frustration by having to push themselves. When a meeting is held to discover why this child, who has been passing up to this point, is failing the sixth grade, everyone scratches their head. They usually do not consider ADD as a possible explanation. They sometimes erroneously assume the presence of a psychological problem as an explanation for the child's failure. They cannot understand why a child who has had ADD in the first five grades was not diagnosed earlier. They also find it hard to understand why the child did not fail earlier.

It is basically very simple. All children are not the same! Some children, with the proper motivation from parents or internal drive, push themselves hard and study long hours. Sometimes the parents help them an inordinate amount of time in order to allow them to pass. This may work for a few years until the child gets to the point that they can no longer study for hours on end without becoming aggravated and frustrated.

I have had many parents tell me that the child can do the work, but they just won't. Teachers are notorious for this phrase. This is a true statement, the child can do the work. No one seems to understand just how difficult it is for them to do the work. An example that I often use is: "Imagine two ditches, each ten feet long and two feet deep. They are exactly alike. However, one was dug with a shovel and the other was dug with a spoon. If you went out into the backyard and pointed at these two ditches and said, "Do not tell me that you cannot dig that ditch with a spoon, there is the proof. You can do it, if you only would." Well, you would be correct, it can be done with a spoon. But you are overlooking how much time and effort it took to dig the ditch with a spoon as opposed to the ditch dug with a shovel. Now, this is like comparing these ADD children with the average child. They can do the work, but they have to push themselves extremely hard. It takes an emotional toll that we may not see until years later. Sometimes, we never know of the effect it has had. Interestingly, one of the most common emotional problems of these children is low self-esteem. This is probably because of the years of failure in the family, at school, and with peer relationships.

You must remember that this disorder is physiological, that is, it is not a psychological problem. However, it does cause emotional problems eventually. It is a real physical problem (neurological).

Just as you cannot cure a broken arm by talking to it, so with ADD, you cannot cure it by counseling either the children or the parents. The only treatment that has proven to be effective is medication. This will also be discused later in the book.

SOCIAL FUNCTIONING

These children are usually seen as being more immature than others. Many of these children are afraid of the dark and some become extremely dependent upon their mothers. Some develop separation anxiety to the point of being afraid to go

to school because they fear their mother will
not come to get them. If they have friends, they
are usually younger and they may even prefer
toys of younger children. Many are selfish, they
lie, and they are dishonest. This is more true
of ADD children with hyperactivity than those
without it.

These children appear to have little awareness
as to how their misbehaviors lead to negative
consequences. This may be hard for most people
to understand, but these children have difficulty
understanding the consequences of their actions.
ADD children accuse other people. Their primary
defense mechanism is projection. They blame
outside influences for their getting into trouble.
This includes parents, teachers, and peers. They
have very little ability to look inside themselves
and see how they have contributed to their plight.
However, many of these children may show genuine
remorse for misbehaviors incurred earlier. This
only confuses the parents more when they notice
that their child is truly sorry about what they
have done. However, this doesn't necessarily curb
the misbehaviors.

These children have few abilities to plan
for the future, therefore, the consequences of
their actions are not likely to be well thought
out. In time, they may be able to recognize their
wrong doing. Unfortunately, it may be too late.

In considering the aforementioned problems,
you may now understand why these children may
have trouble keeping friends. They play too rough,
they blame others, they want to be the boss,
and they throw temper tantrums. Consequently,
friendships are short lived although they may
have gained these friends quite easily.

CHAPTER V

FAMILY DYNAMICS

You must remember that this disorder is hereditary. Therefore, the parents are an extremely important part of the child's environment. It is likely that one of the parents has had the disorder. Because the disorder includes impulsiveness, and a lack of organizational skills, it is important to note that one of the parents may be disorganized and impulsive. Therefore, they will have an impact on the child's emotional environment aside from the problem the child already has with ADD.

Because many of the children with ADD have a high tolerance for pain, are impulsive, and disorganized, it is important to consider the effect this has upon their siblings. The dynamics involved in families with ADD children are extremely important in understanding the effect this disorder has on those who come in contact with the ADD child.

PSYCHIATRIC PROBLEMS

Research shows that the parents of these children are likely to experience depression. An above average contact with the law, alcoholism,

and other drug abuse, is also more common among
these parents. This, many times, makes it very
simple for clinicians to hypothesize that the reason
the child is behaving the way he does, or the
reason he is depressed and cannot make good
grades is because of the behavior of the parents.
All of this seems to make sense. You can look
within the family and see that the parents are
alcoholic or that the parents exhibit behavior
that is out of the ordinary (i.e., temper outburst,
impulsive and over-reactive). Therefore, clinicians
may over-simplify the problem and overlook the
diagnosis of ADD. They instead focus upon the
parents and their role in the child's behavior.
It is true that the parents have an impact upon
the child, but, if the child has ADD, it is unlikely
that the child's behavior is going to substantially
change by dealing with the parents. Remember,
this is a physiological problem. The parents of
ADD children usually have more marital problems
than other parents. It is questionable as to why
this is the case. One explanation could be that
one of the parents has the disorder and is therefore
very difficult to live with. Or, neither have the
disorder, but having a child who does have the
disorder creates havoc. Each parent may blame
the other for not controlling or teaching the child
properly. The mothers of these children are usually
the heavies.

Because they are around the child more often
than the father, the child's misbehavior is seen
as the mother's fault. "The mother must not be
teaching the child properly." After all, when the
father comes home from work and tells the child
to do something, there is little back-talk. The
child complies. If the child minds him, but doesn't
mind the mother, he can only come to one con-

clusion. The mother is too lenient. This method of thinking does seem logical. However, there could be another explanation. I remember an old epigram that states, "If you're from out of town, you must be an expert." Of course we know that this isn't true. But the point is, that the child may see the father as something out of the ordinary. This is due, in part, to the fact that the child spends a great deal of time with the mother and knows what to expect from her. This isn't the case with the father. Therefore, the child may listen a bit more intently to the deep voice of this "secondary" adult. However, if the father were to spend most of his time with the child, he is very likely to experience difficulty in dealing with the child.

I have witnessed this situation many times, the father recognizes the weaknesses and the shortcomings of his wife. Therefore, he is inclined to think that the child doesn't have the problem, but his wife has the problem. Because the mother has put up with negative feedback from the father, perhaps teachers, and other professionals, she is prone to become depressed. Research confirms that the mothers of children with ADD are more likely to be depressed than other parents. Consequently, the mother is usually the one who ends up going for therapy and not the child.

Mothers of these children usually go to their family doctor in order to find out what is wrong with their child. The mother may ask the doctor directly if the child is hyperactive, has a physical problem that would keep him from learning, or an emotional problem that would affect his learning. At this point, we must recognize most pediatricians and family doctors are male. We must also remember that physicians work with numerous problems and they are not necessarily experts on Attention Deficit Disorders. Therefore, they may overlook the child as having this disorder because of their unfamiliarity, or they may tell the mother that they do not have this problem. The physician may, instead, recognize the mother's inclination toward depression. Therefore, the physician may attribute the child's problem to the mother's depression.

I have witnessed this over and over again. Professionals seem to overlook the fact that children can cause depression in parents, especially children with ADD. What complicates the picture is that when the parent brings the child to the pediatrician, he may spend only twenty or thirty minutes with the child. In this amount of time, the child is able to exhibit any behavior he wants. Therefore, the physician may see the child when he's on his best behavior and conclude that there is nothing wrong. When the mother leaves the doctor's office, she is likely to be more depressed than ever. If the physician states that there is no physiological problem, there is little left for her to do except go for counseling.

When considering these situations, it is understandable why the parents, especially the mothers, are more depressed and frustrated than other mothers. They are blamed by everyone around them and feel that no one understands what they go through on a daily basis. This may result in the mother seeking counseling for herself or marital discord may arise. (Research confirms the fact that there is more marital discord among parents of ADD children.)

The mother may end up in therapy and it may help to reduce her depression. However, the problem still remains with the child. Unfortunately, many therapists do not look beyond the depression. They do not see the role that a child with ADD may have played in this person's depression. The mother may even be put on medication at one point, in order to deal with these feelings. I hate to sound cynical, but I have discovered that most people, including clinicians, are unlikely to synthesize background information to discover what the true problem is. The therapist may discover that the child is having problems at home and school and may therefore request family counseling. Again, all of this seems logical. This type of counseling can go on for years. Why? Because the child has physiological problems and no one is addressing the real issue. I find that therapists sometimes psychologize too much. They tend to overlook signs that indicate that the child may have a problem. What they usually do, is look into the mother's background to see if there is some unresolved conflict or personal life experience that may help the therapist understand why the person is depressed. I am not saying that everyone who is depressed has a child with ADD. What I am saying is that the explanation for a parent's depression may be more obvious if a detailed social history of her children is taken. We must remember that children can put stress on any family. Children with ADD are even more likely to put stress on parents.

I have found that it is possible to look into the background of any person and find some experience that could be the focus of intensive therapy. I can psychologize and make an impressive case. Because I am the professional, the patient may "buy into" my explanation. I have found that this is the case with a great number of therapists. I have seen children after they have been in therapy for two years, who have improved very little. I have seen families who have been in therapy for several years who also have had little improvement. The reason, I have found, was due to the fact that the therapist had overlooked the true problems. He had become enmeshed in some sort of family dynamic system and overlooked the simple fact that one of the children had ADD and was disrupting the family. When the child with ADD is treated, there may be an amazing change in the dynamics of the family. Many times, the chaos and hostility subsides.

SIBLINGS

I would now like to discuss siblings of ADD children. Research shows that if one child has ADD the likelihood of their sibling having it is high. This is especially true if the sibling is a male. Remember, this disorder is 10 times more common in males than in females. It is also hereditary. Therefore, it is not unusual to find more than one child in the family who has ADD. Hence, more than one child is likely to be a candidate for medication. When on-lookers discover that two children of the same family are on medication, they are likely to be suspicious of the parents' motives. Most people seem to think that the only reason a child is on medication is so that the parents do not have to put up with the kid's behavior. This type of thinking is common and denotes a lack of understanding about this disorder. Having more than one child on medication also makes a physician uncomfortable. Again, it is not impossible for more than one child of the same parents to have this disorder.

OLDER SIBLINGS WITHOUT ADD

We must remember that living in a family which has a child with ADD creates problems for all members. The effect on an older child who doesn't have ADD is as follows: First of all, the younger sibling who does have ADD is usually difficult to discipline. If the older sibling is put in a situation where he must babysit this child, numerous problems may arise. Think about it. If you're a parent, you recognize what it is to cope with this child. Imagine how difficult it will be for a sibling to deal with this child. The older sibling does not have the patience, experience, or authority that you, the parent, have. Therefore, they are very likely to become frustrated and may even be aggressive toward their younger brother or sister. Research shows that the siblings of ADD children are more depressed than siblings of non-ADD children. This underlines the stress ADD children put upon their siblings. If the older child is held responsible for their younger sibling, quite often it is likely that the older sibling may end up depressed and frustrated.

The older sibling who babysits may sometimes have to use strong language or physical restraint to get the younger child to comply to their demands. When the parents return home, the younger child reports all of the terrible things his sibling did to him. The parents usually end up reprimanding the older child for being too rough. Imagine the frustration of the older sibling when they are caught in the middle like this. The parents sometimes forget how difficult this child is to handle. Consequently, they end up giving the same advice to the older sibling that others have been giving them - - - - "be more patient and understanding."

YOUNGER SIBLINGS WITHOUT ADD

Let us now reverse the situation. Imagine that the older sibling has ADD and the younger one does not. The effect on the younger child who doesn't have ADD is as follows: If the older ADD child is put in charge of the younger one, chaos is sometimes in store. Remembering that ADD children may have a high tolerance for pain, it is likely that the child with ADD, in this case the older child, will be rough in play and in discipline. This is because they don't realize that the younger child has a lower pain tolerance and therefore gets hurt more easily. The older child is also likely to be impulsive. This may result in spontaneous behavior that could be physically and mentally unhealthy for the younger child. Now imagine being the younger child and having to put up with this type of situation over a number of years. The effect could result in low self-esteem, depression, anxiety, and general feelings of inadequacy.

I have witnessed children in this situation. Outsiders, who observe this child may think he has been abused by the parents. Strangely enough, it could be Sibling Abuse. As most parents agree, there will always be fighting between siblings. Many times the parents of these children assume that this is the case, that their discord is merely normal behavior. Unfortunately, this is not the case.

We must remember, that if an ADD child causes a parent to become distressed, it must be twice as distressful for a younger sibling.

FEMALE CHILD WITH ADD BROTHER

The implications here are basically straight-forward and simple. Most boys usually play rougher than girls. A boy who has ADD is likely to be rougher on his sister than most brothers. This may cause the female some emotional problems down the road. This could affect the way she sees other males, and could have an affect on the kind of boyfriend or mate she chooses. (I'm only guessing at this but I feel this can have an impact on her outlook on life.)

AN ONLY CHILD WITH ADD

This situation poses problems for the parents. They have never had a child before, consequently they are not able to compare this child's behavior with that of others. When the parents discuss what kind of problems they have with their child, other parents will say they have the same problems. However, the difference is one of degree. The problems that parents of an ADD child have, are of a more severe degree. These parents may then feel that they are only dealing with "normal childhood behavior". They may conclude that they are not adequate parents and need to work harder. When this only child is adopted, guilt is also part of the parents dilemma. They may conclude that the child had enough problems in his life, and now he's stuck with inadequate par-ents. (Remember, research shows that adopted children are 4 times as likely to have ADD than non-adopted.)

It should be easy to see that the families of these children are more likely to be chaotic than that of the average family. Clinicians who

come in contact with these families are inclined
to see this chaos as the cause of the child's behavior. It is obvious that the family situation
is chaotic and lends support to the conclusion.
Hence, the clinician may start his therapy based
on the assumption that if he changes the chaos
in the family (i.e., the parents behavior), the
child will automatically get better. I must say
that this is the case in some families. This is
not necessarily true when dealing with a child
who has ADD. Remember, this is a physiological
problem, and will require more than rearranging
the environment.

THE PARENTS

At this point I must challenge an old belief
system. This belief system says that parents have
an effect on children but children do not have
an effect on parents. This is why it is always
seen as a parent's problem when a child is not
doing well in some area. Parents are the first
ones to be blamed. Again, I'm not saying that
some parents don't create problems in some instances. But, in families where an ADD child
is present, the child is usually the problem, not
the parents. Unfortunately, casual observers do
not know that the child has ADD. Therefore,
they are probably going to blame the parents
for not controlling their child. Parents have had
other adults say things such as, "If I could have
him for 24 hours, he would learn how to mind."
We must remember the characteristics of a child
with ADD. They are impulsive, have a high tolerance for pain, easily distracted, have a short
attention span, have emotional outbursts, temper
tantrums, and do not respond well to discipline.
It's easy to understand how much stress a parent

must endure when they must cope with a child who has these kinds of problems. These parents, like everyone else, usually believe that the child's functioning is a reflection of the parents' child rearing abilities. Therefore, they are inclined to blame themselves for their child's misbehaviors. It is ironic that these parents are acused of being inadequate and negligent.

I have discovered that these parents are usually more conscientious than the average parent because of the extra effort that they must put forth in order to keep their child in control. These children may always be difficult to handle, even when treated with medication. My point is, that these children may adversely affect the parents emotional state, more than an average child could.

I would now like to discuss the effects the children may have upon the child rearing skills of the parents. All parents usually begin disciplining their children in ways in which their parents used. These techniques may work for most children, but may not be effective with an ADD child. For example: A common method of dealing with negative behavior is to ignore it. The theory is, that the child is seeking attention so you must not reinforce this negative behavior by giving them attention. If you ignore the negative, and reinforce the positive, their behavior will change. This may work with the average child. Unfortunately, ADD children do not respond to this approach. Research indicates that these children respond to negative reinforcement more than positive reinforcement. Parents discover this through practical experience. They discover that the child's behavior may become worse if they use only positive reinforcement. At this point

the parent has to resort to verbal threats or physical discipline. This may, or may not, be effective
over the long term. ADD children are usually
slow in learning about what is and is not proper
behavior. This means that they are inclined to
repeat the same infraction that got them into
trouble only minutes earlier. Therefore, the parent
must repeat the aforementioned sequence of events.
After this scene being repeated a number of times,
the parent may do one of several things:

1. Blow up and severely punish the child.
2. Give up and let him/her do as they wish.
3. Give up on trying to discipline the child
   for every offense and just concentrate
   on the big ones. (i.e., running off without permission, playing with dangerous
   items.)
4. Continue to try to discipline the child
   for every infraction.

Because these children get into more trouble
than other children, the parents usually have to
give up on trying to discipline every infraction.
Over time, the parent, usually the mother, dis-
covers that it is sometimes easier to do things
herself, rather than spend 10 minutes trying to
get the child to do it. The parent may begin to
overlook certain misbehaviors. This may be due
to the fact that they recognize that they are
almost always expressing negative feedback to
the child. They recognize that this could be detrimental to the child's self-concept, so they try
to reduce their negative feedback. The parent
may begin to feel guilty for being so tough on
the child. This guilt may be enhanced if a professional or relative criticizes the parent.

Eventually, parents may finally recognize
what works and what does not. They discover

the initial threats and verbal restrictions do not work with these children. After weeks, months, or even years of trying new approaches, they find out that they must go straight to the methods that work if they want the child to comply. Unfortunately, the methods that seem to work the best are the ones in which the parent has to become angry and make a big scene in order to get the child's attention.

I have been using the word <u>parent</u> for the past few paragraphs instead of designating the mother or father. At this time, I will point out that the mother is the parent who usually deals with the child most often. This is an important point, because it is the mother who experiences the most stress in dealing with the ADD child. Again, research indicates that mothers of ADD children are more likely to become depressed than mothers of non-ADD children.

Now back to the point I was making earlier.

Because the mother sees that she cannot stay on the child all the time, she may start ignoring the "little misbehaviors." A problem between her and her husband may arise when he observes this. In fact, he may start correcting the child for these "little misbehaviors" and actually get results. The child may mind him. This may make him conclude that his wife is not doing her job properly. Instead of accusing her of being too tough, he may accuse her of being too easy. This may become frustrating to the mother because she is now accused of being both too easy and too hard. She may start feeling that either there is actually something wrong with her approach or that others just don't understand with what she must deal on a daily basis. She may have trouble convincing her husband that it would be physically and emotionally impossible to discipline the child for everything he does wrong.

After the parents have spent several years in tolerating this type of behavior, they may find themselves resenting the child. There is a tendency for the parents to become more withdrawn from the child. They may even get to the point of saying that they don't like them. Obviously, this leads to feelings of guilt because they recognize they should not be having these feelings. This is especially true for the mother. Ironically, other people are likely to really enjoy these children. That is, of course, if they only spend short periods of time around them. This is because they are usually energetic, talkative, friendly, and humorous. This may be charming for an hour or two but after months or years, they lose their charm. The parents, especially the mother, may begin protecting themselves emotionally. They do this by reacting to the child as if they are "things" and not people. These children are sometimes emotionally brutal. They may demean the parents or embarrass them by making unusual comments in public places. These children may also refuse parental attempts at showing affection.

If you are an outsider, and observe the parents treatment of these children, you may conclude that the parents are cold, harsh, and do not give the child enough affection. Your conclusion may be correct. However, there is a great deal of information that you are not aware of that would help you better understand the parents' situation.

PARENTS AND PHYSICIANS

Imagine that you are a doctor and a parent comes to you for help with their difficult child. This parent exhibits the aforementioned traits in dealing with the child. Guess what the doctor is inclined to conclude? Yes, he is a human being who will observe the same thing that others observe. Therefore, he is more likely to focus his attention on the parent rather than the child. I have witnessed this on numerous occasions. The doctor may observe the child for 20 to 30 minutes in an office that is unfamiliar to the child. Since this is a doctor's office, the child may be scared. Hence, what the doctor observes is the child being on his best behavior. I am amazed at how many physicians do not take this into consideration when trying to diagnose a child. They seem to discount what the parent, usually the mother, tells them about the child's behavior. Most physicians are male, and I am inclined to think that they see many of these women as neurotic and in need of help. It is understandable why. They observe an upset mother and a relatively calm child in their office. The mother may become more upset if the doctor implies that she is the problem. Some doctors may then refer the parent to a therapist, for counseling.

PARENTS AND THERAPISTS

Believe it or not, this is where the aforementioned scene is repeated again. The therapists will observe the parent, usually the mother, and the child. The mother is likely to show signs of depression, and the child is likely to appear calm or happy go lucky. The therapist may focus on the depression of the mother rather than the misbehavior of the child. He may provide her with child management techniques to help her with her child. This is only done as a side issue, his main focus is on the mother's depression. The child management techniques that were provided to her are usually the very same things that she has already tried. They were not successful. Since he is the professional, she may again attempt these techniques. Parents have told me that when they have told the therapist that what they have suggested will not work, the therapist became indignant. What most therapists may assume is, that these techniques work, but the parent must not be doing them properly. Again, the inclination is to blame the parent for the child's misbehavior.

Although most physicians and therapists may claim to know about ADD, I find that their knowledge is usually incomplete. Therefore, they may overlook this disorder, especially if there are more obvious signs suggesting a problem with the parent.

CHAPTER VI

ADD FROM BIRTH TO ADULTHOOD

We will now examine ADD from infancy into adulthood. Characteristics of the disorder in different stages of life will be discussed.

INFANCY

From birth, ADD children with hyperactivity may show their dislike of being cuddled. Their sleeping patterns may be irregular. They may not need to sleep as long as most children. Some parents have reported that their children liked to be held as you would hold a sack of potatoes with their arms and legs free.

From age two to three, misbehaviors may be noticeable in many of these children. You may start noticing the non-compliance. A parent may have to repeat their instructions quite often before the child obeys. At this time, they are also likely to show their proneness to accidents. They are more likely to have more cuts and bruises at this age. This is probably due to their inability to recognize situations that could result in physical harm.

Many parents may attribute these behaviors to the terrible twos' syndrome. It is important to notice the distinction between the behavior of ADD children and non-ADD children. All children go through the terrible twos', but these children are likely to exhibit more than the average amount of symptoms.

PRE-SCHOOL YEARS

ADD children are likely to come to the attention of professionals at this time, especially if they go to pre-school or kindergarten. This is because staff members are more likely to note that there is something different about this child when compared to other children with whom they deal. Staff members will probably say something vague such as, these children need "psychological" help. They will probably not be able to state that these children have ADD; all they will point out is that something is different about them.

At this age, these children can become problems when in public places. Shopping in a supermarket can be very difficult because they are apt to go out scouting and pull things from the shelves. The parent is placed in an awkward situation and may decide to delay shopping until the child is with a sitter. In pre-school years, the parents may become more concerned because the child does not seem to consider the consequences of his behavior. When the parent looks into the future, they may see hints of what is to come if the child's attitude does not change.

At this age, traditional punishment measures may begin to prove ineffective as a deterrent. When punished, these children may become angry and start having temper tantrums. Unable to see how their behavior contributed to their punishment, they may start blaming their problems on other people, such as playmates, or siblings.

Aggression is sometimes seen at this age. This may not be due to an innate desire to be mean, it may have something to do with their pain tolerance. Since they can tolerate pain much more than other children, they may feel that others can tolerate as much pain as they can. Therefore, they may play rougher than their mates. This could result in them hurting the other children. Consequently, the other children may refuse to play with them.

At this age, they may start taking toys apart or destroying them. These children seem to be very inquisitive and take toys apart just to see how they work. They may or may not be able to put them back together in an operable state. After approximately five years of dealing with this child, the parents may start getting to a point of being "burned out." The mother is most susceptible since she spends more time with the child. It is likely that the mother may start becoming depressed and feeling inadequate, blaming herself for her child's inability to go by the rules.

ENTERING SCHOOL

During the school years, ADD children with hyperactivity are more likely to come to the forefront. At this point in time, parents usually start hearing from the school staff. School personnel may start to develop a negative and judgmental attitude toward the child. Often, the parents are accused of being the cause of their child's

behavior problems. I have found that this is especially the case if they live in a small town where
the background of the parents is known. If the
parents had any type of trouble as a child, adolescent, or adult, it will be remembered and referred
to as proof of their guilt in "ruining" their child.

Many teachers, at this point, may feel that
the child is immature and suggest that they be
retained in a grade until they catch up with their
peers. The reasoning involved here seems logical.
This thinking is, if you wait a year or so, the
child will "mature" enough to be able to function
adequately and they won't have any more problems.
Unfortunately, this is not the case with ADD
children. The immaturity, short attention span,
distractibility, and inability to concentrate for
long periods of time does not usually go away
over a three month summer. Remember, this
is a physiological problem that does not disappear
overnight or in four months. Therefore, holding
the child back a year will not be effective in
"curing" their "immaturity". If the child is already
older than peers, holding them back may increase
their chances of never graduating from high school.
I have seen some of these kids who were fifteen
or sixteen and in the eighth grade. This means
that they will be twenty years old when they
graduate. That is, of course, if they do not fail
another grade.

The appearance of learning disabilities may
become noticeable in the first and second grades.
However, those parents who work with their children hours on end, are likely to compensate for
a learning disability. Consequently, the child may
not come to the attention of the teacher or any
other school personnel because their grades are

satisfactory. Also, children with an above average intelligence may be able to overcome some of these learning difficulties by extra effort. It is okay to exert extra effort, but, if a child has to exert this extra effort over a number of months or years, it could result in their becoming frustrated with school.

At this time, ADD with hyperactivity and ADD without hyperactivity must be separated. ADD children without hyperactivity are not as likely to come to the attention of the school personnel. It must be remembered that all children have a personality and some are more outgoing than others. The same is true of ADD children. Not all of these children are outgoing and rambunctious. Compared to ADD children with hyperactivity, ADD children without hyperactivity will seem very "normal".

An ADD child without hyperactivity may be a model child in the classroom. They may be compliant and reserved, and have no behavioral problems. These children may even become scape goats for others. Consequently, the teachers may start protecting the child. If the child has trouble with the school work, it may be seen as a result of the child's emotional state. The teacher may suspect outside influences such as parental abuse, especially if the child seems meek and withdrawn.

Teachers and other professionals may be appalled when a non-hyperactive child is diagnosed as having ADD. This is because they equate ADD with hyperactivity. Since these children are not "hyper" the diagnosis of ADD seems unwarranted. Many parents trust the teacher's opinion and therefore may not seek the proper treatment for the child (i.e., medication). At this time in the school year, these children may start noticing that they are loners, but not by choice. Others may start leaving them out of the group. There are several reasons for this. It may be because of their silly behavior, their off the wall comments, or their inability to know when to stop a certain behavior. These children may irritate others past the normal limits of most children. As the years go by, their academic performance may or may not decline. This is because all children are different and all parents are different in the way in which they work with their child. As previously stated, those parents who work diligently and long hours with their child are more likely to keep their child from coming to the attention of school personnel. In a way, this is harmful to the child. If he had come to the attention of school officials earlier, he could have been referred for help at an earlier time.

At this time in their lives, these children may start being untrustworthy and engage in petty theft. Many of these children feel that if they want something, they should just take it. Most people may think that the parents are not teaching values to the child. The parents may even feel guilty and blame themselves for not teaching the child properly. It is difficult for people to understand that this behavior is the result of having ADD. These children have a difficult time recognizing the negative consequences of their actions. Since they are impulsive, they act before they think. Teaching these children moral values is very difficult, and takes more repetition than one would expect of the average child.

Throughout childhood, ADD children are likely to continue to exhibit depression. Their self-esteem is also likely to continue declining. This is probably due to the fact that they have been failing in school, social situations, and within the family. These kids may start bragging and lying in order to compensate for their negative feelings. They lie and brag about their achievements in order to look more important in the eyes of other people and themselves. They may actually start believing the lies or exaggerated accomplishments that they tell others. Hence, others may feel that they are on the verge of being out of touch with reality.

Because school becomes a negative factor in their life, truancy may increase. This may be especially the case for junior and high school students. Research shows that many of the kids who are in trouble with the juvenile authorities are very likely to have ADD. Unfortunately, many are not diagnosed as having ADD, and consequently receive the wrong treatment. They are usually diagnosed as conduct disorders.

Sometimes these children will be in special education classes under the label of emotionally disturbed. They may not qualify for special education based on their intelligence and achievement scores. They usually score too high in these areas to qualify for placement. Therefore, the label of emotionally disturbed must be used in order to provide an educational placement for these kids.

Because they are getting older and their tastes start to change, disruption of the family life may become more prevalent. When they were six or seven years old, their non-compliance probably related to not wanting to go to bed, refusing to eat, or breaking toys. Now that they are in the teen years, their desires and wants become much different. They may start staying out a little later, having temper outbursts, and perhaps scaring the parents with threats of violence or of self-destruction.

ADOLESCENCE

It must be remembered that these years are the most difficult for all humans. When another adverse factor is introduced into a person's life at this time, the child is likely to experience more confusion and frustration than the "average" child. This is the case with ADD children. Life is more confusing to them than it is for others their age. Therefore, the so called "normal" stages of rebellion and depression may be more pronounced with these adolescents.

Parents become frustrated with all teenagers. However, the parents of ADD children are likely to experience more frustration than others. The ADD adolescent therefore, experiences a great deal of negative feedback from the parents whose tolerance level has been pushed beyond the limits. The adolescent's continued school failure ensures negative feedback from both parents and teachers. Their self-esteem may plummet to an all time low due to the aforementioned. These adolescents do not see themselves as very smart because they are usually failing some classes.

Research shows that depression is very common among adolescents with ADD. (More so than that of non-ADD adolescents.) They usually have low self-esteem and do not expect much from the future. Their self-confidence is at an all time

low. Research also shows that in the later adolescent periods, say fifteen or sixteen, alcohol abuse
is much more common than in the average teenager. At this point, I would like to give an explanation as to why I think this happens.

The first thing you must remember is that
the most successful treatment for this disorder
is medication. This is because ADD is a physical
problem. It is a neurological problem indicating
some sort of chemical imbalance in the brain.
The most effective treatment is medication. Now,
suppose that a child has had this disorder for
fifteen years and hasn't been treated. At fifteen
years of age, they may begin experimenting with
things like alcohol, marijuana, or other substances.
Unfortunately, when an ADD child experiences
alcohol, it is likely that he will get a good feeling.
Why? Primarily because he has just experienced
"treatment" for his disorder. He has medicated
himself. The medication, (i.e., alcohol) has in
effect, treated the ADD and made him feel less
confused, a little more organized, and confident.

After such a positive experience, it may
be difficult to convince this child that alcohol
is bad for them. To them, they feel better when
they drink. In actuality, they do feel better. Unfortunately, the alcohol may help them feel better,
but it is the wrong medication for treating ADD.
Consequently, they must continually increase
the dosage in order to get the same effects that
they experienced the first time they drank. As
they increase the amount over a period of time,
it will start having an adverse effect on other
parts of the body.

On the other hand, if they had been medicated
with the right medicine, the amount they would

have to take would be very low and it would not have to be constantly increased. Once the appropriate level is obtained, there is no need for an increase. Research shows that ADD children who were treated with medication, were shown to abuse alcohol and drugs much <u>less</u> than other adolescents. (Note: This means that they are <u>less likely</u> to abuse drugs than other people in general, not just ADD children who were not treated.)

Past research indicates that ADD children who are <u>not</u> treated, are likely to abuse alcohol and other drugs more than the average teenager. A major point is, that if they are treated when they are <u>young</u>, they are less likely to abuse drugs. The older they get, the harder it is to treat them successfully.

In adolescence, sexual urges arise. This is the case with all adolescents. I have discovered that adolescents with ADD are likely to experience their sexual urges in a more intense fashion.

This means that when they experience sexual excitement, their feelings may be beyond that of the average adolescent. When you combine this trait with the other traits of ADD adolescents (i.e., impulsiveness, not considering the consequences of their actions), sexual acting out is likely. Therefore, unwanted pregnancies may arise among ADD adolescents. Because these adolescents are immature and irresponsible, they are usually unable to take care of a child. Consequently, the child must either be given up for adoption or aborted.

Research indicates that adoptive children are 4 times more likely to have ADD than non-adoptive children. I believe the aforementioned scenario is the explanation as to why this occurs. I have worked with a number of adolescent females who had ADD and became pregnant. They had to give the child to an adoption agency. Since the disorder is hereditary, there is a good chance that the child will have ADD.

I also see the potential for suicide as being a big problem among ADD adolescents. There are many factors which contribute to this. First of all, consider the fact that they have had the disorder since birth. If they weren't treated, it is probable that they have attained a low self-image. This low self-image was probably due to them having had difficulty in achieving at school, fitting in with peers, or getting along with parents. They may have had difficulty in all three areas. As most professionals will tell you, a low self-image is one of the traits among those who are suicidal. When this is considered with other traits previously mentioned (i.e., impulsiveness, intense emotionality), the scene is set for suicidal ideation. I have worked with numerous ADD adolescents who were sucidal. They felt as if they were unable to do anything well.

In connection with suicide, we must also remember that car accidents are one of the biggest killers of American teenagers. Since ADD adolescents are more reckless, crave excitement, and do not anticipate the consequences of their actions, they are more likely to be involved in auto accidents than other teens. (Numerous professionals feel that some fatal auto accidents are disguised suicides.)

ADULTHOOD

In adulthood, the problems that they face are of a different type. Because they did not perform well in school, it is unlikely that they will go to college. The requirements of concentrating and paying attention are too demanding. After high school, they probably do not want to experience the frustration of academia any longer.

Problems that began in adolescence may continue. For example, alcohol and drug abuse may continue or increase. These individuals are prone to keep on the move. They usually gravitate toward jobs that allow them the freedom of behavior that they enjoy. They may have trouble keeping a job for a long period of time due to their nomadic need of moving on to greener pastures.

As adults, impulsiveness, restlessness, and a short attention span may continue to be a problem. If they get married, they may have trouble being a faithful mate. If they have temper outbursts, they could end up being abusive to both their mates and children. Research shows that divorce is common among these individuals. Illegal activities and incarceration is shown to be more common with these individuals than those who did not have ADD.

At the end of this book, adult case studies will be presented. Also, my next book will be more comprehensive on the adult who has had ADD.

CHAPTER VII

EVALUATION

First it must be emphasized that evaluation of these children is difficult. There is no one psychological test, blood test, neurological test, or achievement test that will tell you whether or not this child has ADD. One of the most important factors in diagnosing a child correctly is having someone who is experienced in dealing with this disorder. Many professionals are going to say that they have experience with this disorder, but I have discovered that their knowledge is usually incomplete. The phrase, "a little knowledge is a dangerous thing," is appropriate when considering the familiarity of professionals with ADD.

The information I am giving you about ADD will probably put you ahead of most professionals in terms of knowledge about ADD. This especially includes the ability to diagnose it. If you are the parent, you know more about your child than a professional. If the professional doesn't ask the right questions or observe the child in his normal mode of behavior, it is likely that he will not be able to diagnose the child properly.

I am saying that you must trust your judgment and challenge your professional. After you learn

more about ADD, you will be able to ask intelligent questions. If the professional cannot answer
your questions to your satisfaction, I would suggest
that you go to another. I have witnessed numerous
children who have been misdiagnosed by pediatricians and psychiatrists. Therefore, do not necessarily be impressed by the credentials. They are
human beings first, and professionals second.

The consequences of overlooking a child with
ADD could be severe. It may take several years
for the results to become evident. Adolescence
is usually when the negative consequences become
most evident.

Therefore, if you suspect your child has ADD,
I suggest you not give up on treatment. This may
mean that you will make a lot of enemies with
doctors, therapists, teachers, and counselors,
but the child's future is worth it.

The information in this book will not totally
enable you to diagnose your child as having ADD,
however, you will have as much information at
your fingertips as most professionals. Perhaps
more. So, I suggest that you go to a professional,
but be prepared with questions. This will force
him to expose his knowledge, or lack of knowledge
of ADD.

Therefore, this section of the book is used
as a guideline. It is what I use and has been very
effective. You must remember someone's personal
judgment and personal contact with the child
cannot be duplicated in a book.

It is important that the person who conducts
the evaluation be able to direct you to a neurolo-

gist, pediatrician, etc. In other words, one person needs to have the final say in direction of treatment. If not, you will get 5 different opinions and become confused. I have found that someone's credentials are important, but not as important as their personality. There are good ditch diggers and there are bad ditch diggers. There are good attorneys and there are bad attorneys. There are good medical doctors and bad medical doctors. My point is, that someone's credentials alone should not impress you. Talk with them, listen to them, see if they seem to make sense. If they are "blowing smoke" or they do not have time for you, you must decide whether or not you want to use them. Again, do not assume that anyone you go to is knowledgeable about ADD. Question and challenge them. Remember, they work for you.

Evaluation consists of a number of things. Here is a list of the techniques used. They will be presented in this order, in more detail.

- Parent Questionnaire
- Teacher Questionnaire
- Medical History of Child
- Social History of Child
- Medical History of Parents (Brief)
- Social History of Parents
- Observation of Child
- Clinical Interview of Parents

Other Techniques:

- Achievement/Educational/Psychological Testing
- Neurological Screening
- Allergy Tests

- Auditory Test
- Visual Test
- Dental Check-up

PARENT/TEACHER QUESTIONNAIRE

The following questionnaires were developed by Dr. Keith Conners. It is important to get every item answered. However, only 10 items on each of the questionnaires is pertinent in diagnosing ADD. Some of the other items will inform you about other aspects of the child's behavior. They may also contradict what has been checked on some of the "10" items. This is when you must use your judgment in determining the true description of the child.

PARENT'S QUESTIONNAIRE	Not at all	Just a little	Pretty much	Very much
1. Picks at things (nails, fingers, hair, clothing).				
2. Sassy to grown-ups.				
3. Problems with making or keeping friends.				
4. Excitable, impulsive.				
5. Wants to run things.				
6. Sucks or chews (thumb, clothing, blankets).				
7. Cries easily or often.				
8. Carries a chip on his shoulder.				
9. Daydreams.				
10. Difficulty in learning.				
11. Restless in the "squirmy" sense.				
12. Fearful of new situations, new people, new places, (going to school).				
13. Restless, always up and on the go.				
14. Destructive.				
15. Tells lies or stories that aren't true.				
16. Shy.				
17. Gets into more trouble than others same age.				
18. Speaks differently from others same age (baby talk, stuttering, hard to understand).				

	Not at all	Just a little	Pretty much	Very much
19. Denies mistakes or blames others.				
20. Quarrelsome.				
21. Pouts and sulks.				
22. Steals.				
23. Disobedient or obeys but resentfully.				
24. Worries more than others (about being alone, illness, or death).				
25. Fails to finish things.				
26. Feelings easily hurt.				
27. Bullies others.				
28. Unable to stop a repetitive activity.				
29. Cruel.				
30. Childish or immature (wants help he shouldn't need, clings, needs constant reassurance).				
31. Distractibility or attention span a problem.				
32. Headaches.				
33. Mood changes quickly and drastically.				
34. Doesn't like or doesn't follow rules or restrictions.				
35. Fights constantly.				
36. Doesn't get along well with brothers and sisters.				

	Not at all	Just a little	Pretty much	Very much
37. Easily frustrated in efforts.				
38. Distrubs other children.				
39. Basically an unhappy child.				
40. Problems with eating (poor appetite, up between bites).				
41. Stomach aches.				
42. Problems with sleep (can't fall asleep, up too early, up in the night).				
43. Other aches and pains.				
44. Vomiting or nausea.				
45. Feels cheated in family circle.				
46. Boasts and brags.				
47. Lets self be pushed around.				
48. Bowel problems (frequently loose, irregular habits, constipation).				

TEACHER'S QUESTIONNAIRE

	Not at all	Just a little	Pretty much	Very much
1. Restless in the "squirmy" sense.				
2. Makes inappropriate noises when he shouldn't.				
3. Demands must be met immediately.				
4. Acts "smart" (impudent or sassy).				
5. Temper outbursts and unpredictable behavior.				
6. Overly sensitive to criticism.				
7. Distractibility or attention span a problem.				
8. Disturbs other children.				
9. Daydreams.				
10. Pouts and sulks.				
11. Mood changes quickly and drastically.				
12. Quarrelsome.				
13. Submissive attitude toward authority.				
14. Restless, always "up and on the go."				
15. Excitable, impulsive.				
16. Excessive demands for teacher's attention.				
17. Appears to be unaccepted by group.				
18. Appears to be easily led by other children.				
19. No sense of fair play.				

	Not at all	Just a little	Pretty much	Very much
20. Appears to lack leadership.				
21. Fails to finish things that he starts.				
22. Childish and immature.				
23. Denies mistakes or blames others.				
24. Does not get along well with other children.				
25. Uncooperative with classmates.				
26. Easily frustrated in efforts.				
27. Uncooperative with teacher.				
28. Difficulty in learning.				

Each of the traits is scored from 0 to 3 as follows: Not at all = 0, Just a little = 1, Pretty much = 2, Very much = 3. The ten phrases and their numbers on the rating forms are as follows:

	Parent #	Teacher #
• Excitable, impulsive	4	15
• Difficulty in learning	10	28
• Restless in the "squirmy" sense	11	1
• Restless, always up and on the go	13	14
• Fails to finish things	25	21
• Childish or immature	30	22
• Distractibility or attention span a problem	31	7
• Easily frustrated in efforts	37	26
• Mood changes quickly and drastically	33	*
• Denies mistakes or blames others	19	*
• Disturbs other children	**	8
• Demands must be met immediately	**	3

(* This item appears only on the Parent Form; ** This item appears only on the Teacher Form.)

The Hyperkinesis Index is derived simply by totaling the scores of the appropriate ten items on each form. The numerical range of the Index is 0 to 30, with a higher score indicating a greater degree of hyperactivity as judged by a parent or teacher. For research purposes, a total score of at least 36 points on the combined parent and teacher indices (with a teacher's score of at least 18 points) was necessary for a child's inclusion in a basic study group.

In practice, these forms have been found to be useful rating tools when completed at approximately three to six week intervals. It is suggested that shorter intervals be employed whenever the Hyperkinesis Index is used to assess the outcome of altered or newly introduced therapeutic regimes.

Dr. Keith Connors is a Professor of Psychiatry and Neurology and Director of the Laboratory of Behavioral Medicine at Children's Hospital. He was a Rhodes Scholar and holds a doctoral degree in psychology with primary interest in psychopharmacology of childhood, childhood psychopathology, and developmental psychophysiology.

The information on the Parent/Teacher Questionnaires was reprinted by permission of Dr. Keith Conners.

SCORING THE QUESTIONNAIRE

To summarize what was said earlier.

1. Add up the scores of the 10 items on the parent questionnaire.
2. Add up the scores of the teacher questionnaire.
3. Add the two scores together. If the score is 36 or above, there is a high probability that this child has ADD and could benefit from treatment.
4. Scores that are above 30 should raise some serious questions as to whether or not the child has the disorder. The reason being, is that the average child will not usually obtain such a high score. This high score indicates the need for a more in depth investi-

gation and questioning of the parent or teacher.

5. If you only have access to one set of scores, and it is a borderline score, this will also require a more in depth look at the child. (A score of 18 would be borderline, but a score of 15 is sometimes indicative of some sort of problem and warrants a closer investigation.)

6. If more than one teacher's questionnaire is involved, it may require more thought than usual. They may have totally opposite scores. You have to find out why the scores are so different. Sometimes a teacher will not want to answer the questions, so they may just mark them without giving any thought to the accuracy. If a teacher likes a child, they may mark them favorably. They may think that this is helpful to the child, but it is not. The same thing is true for teachers who do not like a particular child. They may make them look worse than they are. In any event, it may take some digging to find what is an accurate score.

7. Trust the parents score. They are usually aware of their child. You must be careful because they could also be miscalculating the child's behavior.

Remember, evaluating a child consists of more than these two questionnaires. Try not to base your decision on the results of only one methodology.

MEDICAL/SOCIAL HISTORY

1. Any physical problems during pregnancy?
2. Was pregnancy full term?
3. Type of delivery:_____.

4. Any problems with delivery or immediately after birth?
5. Is child adopted?

Please indicate if child has experienced any of the following:

NO   YES   AGE

1. Seizures
2. Hearing Impairment
3. Painful or Irregular Menses
4. Fainting Spells
5. Periods of Unconsciousness
6. Severe Headaches
7. Frequent Ear Trouble
8. Vision Problems
9. Head Injury
10. Asthma
11. Loss or Gain of Weight
12. Episodes of prolonged high (103) fever
13. Short of Breath
14. Female Disease or Disorder
15. Bed Wetting
16. Bad Appetite
17. Need less sleep than others
18. Move around a lot in their sleep
19. Liked to be held, cuddled
20. Take toys apart
21. Accident prone
22. More Doctors' Visits than usual

NO   YES   AGE

23. Do they wander away
    from the house
24. Difficulty in finding
    Babysitters

If any of the above were answered yes, please
describe further:_____

_____

_____

SCHOOL AGE CHILDREN

These are some areas in which your attention
must focus for older children:

FIVE TO SEVEN YEARS OLD:
A. Has anyone ever suggested that your child
   is "hyper"?
B. Do they have more trouble coloring between
   the boundaries of coloring books than others?
C. Do teachers complain that they are immature
   for their age?
D. Do teachers suggest that they be held back
   a year in order to mature?
E. Do the teachers complain that the child day-
   dreams and gets up out of his seat more
   often than other children?
F. Does the child seem to have more drastic
   mood swings than other children? Do they
   get angry easily? Are their feelings hurt
   easily?

SEVEN TO TEN YEARS OLD:
A. Do the teachers complain that the child does
   not finish his work?
B. Does the child get in more trouble than others
   their age?

C. Are their grades borderline or less?
D. Have teachers suggested that perhaps your child is hyperactive?
E. Have teachers suggested testing to determine if your child would qualify for Special Education?
F. Has your child been tested for Special Education placement, but scored too high to qualify?

TEN TO TWELVE YEARS OLD:
All of the previously stated problems, but they are more pronounced, i.e.:
A. They are becoming behavior problems in school and being sent to the office.
B. They refuse to complete their work or do not even try to do it.
C. They do the work at home, but do not turn it in at school. Yet, they may swear that they turned it in and blame the teacher for losing it.
D. At the end of the year the unaccounted for homework previously mentioned is found at the bottom of their school lockers.
E. Because they are making poor grades, they gravitate toward other persons who do poorly in school.
F. They seem to have trouble understanding some abstract concepts.
G. They seem to lack "common sense."

ADOLESCENCE (12 AND UP):
A. Do they skip school often?
B. Are they involved in illegal behaviors?
C. Are they involved in drugs/alcohol?
D. Do they abuse inhalants (i.e., gasoline, glue, liquid paper)?
E. Are they not turning in their homework, and talking of quitting school?

F. Are they more disorganized than others?
G. Do they seem depressed often?
H. Do they seem sexually promiscuous.?
I. Are they cruel or void of empathy for others?
J. Do they have trouble keeping friends with "desirable" peers?

MISCELLANEOUS QUESTIONS:
A. Has he/she ever repeated a grade?
B. Do they have any learning disabilities?
C. Have they been in Special Education classes?
D. What is child's feelings toward school?
E. What is child's feelings toward authority figures?
F. Does child prefer younger friends or older?
G. Are they a follower or a leader?
H. How do they react in groups?
I. How do they act in the super market?
J. Was child diagnosed as having epilepsy?
K. Has child been on any medication?
L. How do they respond to caffeine?
M. Have they always had poor handwriting?

MEDICAL/SOCIAL HISTORY OF PARENTS

This part of the evaluation is IMPORTANT because this disorder is hereditary. Therefore, finding out something about the background of the parents is extremely important. Research shows that the background of the father is more important than the background of the mother, although this is not always the case. This disorder is hereditary and seems to come more from the males side than from the females (it can come from either side).

Ask the following:
1. Is there a history of alcohol, drug abuse,

or illegal activities on the father's or mother's side of the family?
2. Is there a history of school difficulties?
3. Is there a history of mood swings?
4. Is anyone adopted?
5. Does this child resemble anyone in the family in terms of behavior?

It may be necessary to ask some of the same questions that were listed previously.

OBSERVATIONAL METHODS

Although you may be able to get some information from a child by observing them directly, it is important to observe the child in his home setting or in the school setting. These children may appear to be different when they are in a different environment. It is important to note the difference between this child's behavior and that of others. You want to determine whether or not there is a difference in their method of play. Are they rougher than other children, do they get mad easier, and are they bossier?

OTHER TECHNIQUES

PSYCHOLOGICAL TESTS
As previously stated there is no psychological test that will tell you whether or not this child has ADD. However, it is sometimes helpful to request testing from the school system to see if the child qualifies for special education placement. You can get this testing by going to an outside source, but the school system will do it for nothing. Therefore, I would suggest that you talk to the school counselor and ask for testing to see if your child qualifies for special education

placement. He may try to talk you out of it, but you have the right of requesting such testing. Especially if there is a strong indication that your child may have a problem. They will give your child a battery of achievement tests and an I.Q. test. This will tell you their weaknesses in reading, mathematics, and other areas.

I must warn you that some children with ADD perform well on these tests. Consequently, they are unlikely to qualify for special educational placement based solely on the results of these tests. The school personnel may tell you that there is absolutely no way that this child can be put in special classes because they do not qualify under regulation so and so. Do not believe it. If your child is doing poorly in school, or struggling, you have the right to request special help. You may have to go beyond the school board, but you have a right to see that your child receives help. Remember, schools were developed for children not vice versa.

Needless to say, these tests are not necessarily the best way to determine whether or not a child has ADD. However, it is important that you request this testing as soon as you suspect a problem.

NEUROLOGICAL SCREENING
Research shows that less than 5% to 6% of ADD children have an EEG show any signs of neurological impairment. This doesn't mean that you should not have one done. If your child is having trouble, you may be interested to see whether or not there is a problem. What I am saying is, that you should not expect a definite YES or NO in reference to whether or not your child has ADD based on a neurological exam.

ALLERGY TESTS

Research shows that a large proportion of these children have allergies and asthma. You may want to have these tests ran because they can sometimes account for <u>some</u> of the activity level of the child. You may want to treat this before you move on to other treatments. Again, there is a high probability that the child will have allergies. Therefore, do not conclude that this will solve the problem if treatment is initiated.

AUDITORY/VISUAL TESTS

Many ADD children exhibit characteristics which make you think that something is wrong with their hearing. It would be worthwhile to determine whether or not there truly is a hearing problem.

ADD children have trouble concentrating. If they are in need of glasses, they may exhibit similar symptoms. Their difficulty in focusing on information on the board or reading, may be misinterpreted as concentration problems. Therefore, it is worthwhile to get their eyes checked.

DENTAL EXAM

If a child has a nerve exposed or other dental problems which irritate the nerves, it may cause a restlessness that may be misinterpreted as hyperactivity. The child may have a high enough pain tolerance that he does not complain enough to warrant the concern of the parent. In any case, it is best to give them an examination to rule this out.

I know it sounds like I am asking the parents to spend a lot of time and money in order to diagnose ADD. Actually, I am giving you more information than you need. I personally suggest the following methods of evaluation.

1. Parent/Teacher Questionnaire.
2. Medical/Social History of Child.
3. History of parents.
4. Observation of child.
5. Neurological screening (occasionally).
6. Educational testing.

I have found that you can usually determine whether or not your child has ADD by using these techniques.

CHAPTER VIII

TREATMENT

There are several different types of treatment methods. I will list all of them, in order of importance. In other words, the most important will come first, followed by the next most important. I am equating the terms important with effective. The effectiveness of the treatment methods was determined through a review of the research. I did not personally do the research, but I did investigate it thoroughly. I must also say that, based on empirical evidence, I have found these same treatment methods to be effective and would list them in the same order of importance.

A
MEDICATION

Please note that I am not a medical doctor. I will be discussing medication and the brain, so I want you to know that my information comes from the research articles listed in the back of the book. I recognize that some experts in one of these fields may cringe when they read some of my explanations, but I feel that these illustrations are appropriate for the lay person.

The _most_ effective treatment for ADD is medication. There are many people who have a different opinion. Unfortunately, opinions are sometimes treated as _fact_. Research shows that all other forms of treatment mentioned are not as effective as medication. In fact, they are not even close. Of course you can always point to a few exceptional cases to support your opinion. This is, of course, why they are considered exceptional. In other words, some children will improve by using other methods, but very few in comparison to the use of medication. The research is abundant on this issue. The results are quite clearly in favor of medication. This is a _fact_.

ADD is a chemical imbalance in the brain. Hence, it is physiological, not psychological or environmental. Remember, it is hereditary. Common sense should dictate that the only thing that will help a disorder that is a chemical imbalance is something that will balance the chemical. Research indicates that medication apparently provides this balance. Just as you cannot cure a broken arm by counseling, you cannot cure ADD with counseling or other methods which focus on events outside of the person. Unfortunately, therapists usually focus upon the emotional or behavioral problems of these children through counseling. Yes, these children may have these problems, but if a correct diagnosis was made, the therapist should realize that the disorder (ADD) contributed to these problems. Therefore, you should first treat the "physiological" problem (ADD) before you address the emotional/behavioral problems. Unfortunately, the underlying, hard to diagnose ADD is often overlooked, while the easy to see and easy to diagnose emotional/behavioral problems become the focus of treatment.

I am not saying that the other methods of treatment, especially child management techniques, should not be used. I am saying that you must treat the problems in the correct order. Otherwise, treatment is unlikely to be successful. This is why some children stay in therapy for years but show little improvement. They are being <u>mistreated</u>. If you were to take this book to your child's therapist and tell him you feel that ADD is the problem, he would probably give you some sort of explanation as to how your child does have symptoms that <u>appear</u> to be similar to characteristics of ADD, but these symptoms are caused by other factors. If he has seen your child for a number of months or years, it is unlikely that he is going to admit that he has misdiagnosed your child. No one likes to admit a mistake, especially after he has charged the parents several thousand dollars for the wrong treatment.

Overlooking or mistreating a child with ADD can have a devastating impact on their future. Research indicates that as adults, these people have more trouble functioning in our society than others. Research also indicates that they are prone to alcohol and other drug abuse. They are also inclined to become involved in illegal activities to the point of being incarcerated. In fact, prisons contain numerous adults who have ADD, but were never treated or diagnosed at an earlier age.

The sad thing is, these peoples lives may have been much different if they had been treated. Knowing this causes me great anguish. I tend to blame my profession for these people turning out like this. In essence the counselors, psychologists, and physicians who treated these people when they were children, are partly to blame for their plight. If they had diagnosed and treated them properly, things may have been different.

Fear of putting a child on medication is a common concern of parents. Most people assume that the reason a child is placed on medication is in order to drug them so that they are easier to handle. They see medication as being prescribed for the parents' benefit and not the child's. They are wrong.

Remember, ADD is a chemical imbalance (a physiological problem). Medication is given to the child in order to treat this problem. The problem most people have, is understanding how treating a chemical imbalance can have anything to do with a child's talking back, fighting, not minding, or forgetting things. I will try to explain the connection.

Again, I am not a medical doctor, chemist, or brain specialist. I will try to explain, in an unsophisticated manner, the connection between the aforementioned. My explanation is not scientifically precise, so those of you who are the experts in this field, please do not be offended.

First of all, there are millions of neurons in the brain. These neurons store information and are responsible for relaying information. These neurons do not touch. Between each neuron is a chemical called a neurotransmitter. Some researchers feel that this is the chemical that causes the problem for ADD children. This chemical is responsible for relaying information from one neuron to another. If this chemical is not "effective," the information or message that is being sent may not be passed properly. The messages that I am speaking of, consist of everyday activities in which we indulge. When you get angry and kick the cat, these messages (impulses) are transmitted by neurons. When you think about quitting your job, but first decide to discuss it with your spouse, these messages (impulses) are transmitted by neurons. When you get mad at someone and think about hitting them, but choose instead to talk, these messages (impulses) are transmitted by neurons.

My point is, that almost everything you do is related to some kind of chemical reaction in the brain. Now, the aforementioned are examples which usually indicate that nothing is wrong with the chemical that relays information.

Imagine, if you will, that a 6 year old child has the impulse to go down the block to see what is happening. This child has a problem with the chemical (Neurotransmitter) that relays these impulses. Therefore, the impulse may be acted upon without considering other information such as: Did mom tell me to stay in the backyard (10 times)? Could I be in danger by walking across the street alone? Will I be punished severely for disobeying? Because the child lacks impulse control, they are not likely to consider all of this information. They have an impulse and they act on it. Hence, impulsiveness! (NOTE: All kids do this, but ADD kids do this more often than most.)

I gave this illustration in order to draw a picture of how something like a chemical imbalance can affect the behavior of a child. Most people have trouble seeing the connection between the two. Therefore, they have trouble understanding how medication can help a child who is a behavior problem. Please note that medication does not always stop these problems. A child with ADD is still likely to be a bit more difficult to handle than the average child. I do hope that my crude illustrations get the major point across.

To summarize, the medication provides the chemical balance that is needed. It improves the child's ability to concentrate, think before he acts, and reduces his tendency toward becoming distracted by external stimuli.

I will now give you the medication and dosage levels that physicians recommend. Again, I am not a medical doctor. The following information was gathered from several sources which are listed in the back of the book. The authors of which, are medical doctors.

It is important to note that the type of medication used for a person beyond puberty is different than that of a child. I will separate these by age.

6 YEARS TO PUBERTY

NAME	BEGINNING DOSE	AVERAGE DAILY DOSE
Methylphenidate (Ritalin)	5mg before meals. Gradual increases of 5 – 10 mg/week.	1. 10 – 40 mg (20 mg or less is usually enough) 2. 2 – 3 times per day. With time release, can give all morning.
D-Amphetamine (Dexedrine)	5 mg 1 or 2 times/day raised by 5 mg/week until proper level.	1. 5 – 15 mg/day
Pemoline (Cylert)	37.5 mg. Increase by 18.75 week till proper dose.	1. 56.25 – 75.0 mg/day 2. Give dose 1 time per day (morning)

PUBERTY AND ADULTS

NAME	BEGINNING DOSE	AVERAGE DAILY DOSE
Imipramine (Tofranil)	25 mg/night increase by 25 mg every 10 – 14 days	1. 75 – 150 mg 2. Split dosage. As dosage increases, give part in morning and part at bedtime (or 12 hours apart)

1. ADMINISTRATION

It is extremely important that the proper medication be given. I am amazed at how many physicians do not tell the parents to change the child's medication when they get into puberty. The three medications given to children are commonly referred to as "Speed". This may sound strange, giving "Speed" to a child with these problems. However, this medication has a paradoxical effect on children. In other words, it slows them down and allows them to concentrate. It has the "speeding" effect on those in puberty or above. Hence, if a child stays on this beyond puberty, it could increase the problems instead of decrease them. Also, one medication may not work, while another one will. Do not assume that there is no hope if medication is tried and it does not work. You may have to try all three medications before positive results are seen. You must also remember that there are a portion of these children who do not respond to medication. Therefore, some 20% - 30% of these children will have to be treated in other ways.

It is important to note the times of administration of the dosage. For example: the reason for giving Ritalin before meals is because the effects will not be as positive if given after meals. I have witnessed many parents that have been giving the child a heavy dosage with little results. I have then discovered that the reason that they do not get results is because they give the medication after the child has eaten.

The reason they do this is because the child is more likely to eat if he takes the medicine after his meal. The medication does reduce children's appetites but it may as well not be given if it isn't given properly.

It may be necessary to try different dosage times for your child. Since all children respond differently to medication, your child may function well when given the medicine after meals. This is something that you may have to discuss with your doctor.

Although your medical doctor is a professional and is supposed to know proper dosages and when to increase, I have found that many are not that familiar with this part of the treatment. Consequently, a physician may do one of two things: he may start out with the correct dosage, but not increase at the proper time. This will result in the parent witnessing progress in the beginning, but will not see this progress continue unless the medication is increased appropriately. Or two, the physician may start out with too high a dosage and this may make the child look like a zombie. I have seen parents who have taken their child off medication because of this very thing. The unfortunate thing is, that they may conclude that they do not want their child on medication, especially if they are going to look drugged all the time. Consequently, they may seek another form of help and discount the effectiveness of medicine.

It must also be pointed out that even when the proper dosage is administered, there may be a few days when the child is more sleepy than usual. This should not frighten the parents because this is a normal reaction. It takes time for the medication to build up in the system and for the child's metabolism to get adjusted to this dosage level. As the body adjusts, you will no longer see drowsiness.

If your child is placed on medicine, please note the chart regarding the maximum dosage levels. If you feel that the dosage level is too high, then it would be good for you to confront your physician. I have discovered that pharmacists usually know more about medication and dosage levels than most physicians. Therefore, it may be a good idea to talk to your pharmacist about the side effects and effectiveness of certain medicines.

2. THINGS TO WATCH FOR

a. There are possible side effects from any medication that a child receives. Ask your physician what these are. Some of the known side effects of the medications mentioned for children who are pre-pubescent are: suppressed appetites, weight loss, restlessness for the first three or four days of the medication, or difficulty in sleeping for two or three days. Strangely enough, it seems that children who have had good appetites before they started taking medication have a lower appetite after taking it. I have witnessed children who have bad appetites before they start taking medication, but better appetities afterward. Obviously, there is no way to tell how each child will respond to a given medication.

b. All children are different, therefore, one medication may work for one child while another may not.

c. Remember, during the first three or four days, the medication is getting into their bloodstream. Therefore, what you see, such as more restlessness or poor appetite, may not be long term. The parents, after witnessing their child being sleepy for two or three days, and looking drugged, sometimes decide to take the child off of medication. This is a mistake. After the medication gets into the bloodstream, the benefits far outweigh the risks.

3. PUBERTY AND BEYOND

Again, I am not a medical doctor, but based on my experience, it is important to understand some of the following things. Just because a person is a medical doctor does not assure you that they understand the medication and the proper distribution of that medication. I have found that many pharmacists are more familiar with the medication than the medical doctors. Therefore, I would like to list the following things to look for:

a. Medication must be prescribed first at a low dosage and slowly increased every seven or ten days until the proper dosage is reached.

b. Medication is based on body weight. If a child's weight increases or decreases by 5 - 10 lbs., it may be necessary to change the dosage level. Therefore, what is appropriate for a child who is ninety pounds may not be appropriate if he loses 10 lbs. Therefore, body weight should be monitored.

c. If a person has had a history of medication usage, it may be necessary for their dosage to be higher than normal. Some people have a higher tolerance than others.

NOTE: Their are always possible long term side effects of medication. Read the Physicians Desk Reference about the medicine. Please remember that there are also possible long term side effects of not treating a child who has ADD. The benefits and risks must be weighed before a decision is made.

B
BEHAVIORAL MANAGEMENT TECHNIQUES

For the past few years there have been many behavioral management programs for all types of problems. These behavioral management techniques are adequate and I will not waste your time by mentioning them again. I find that when drug management is used first, these behavioral management techniques are more effective. I will give a few broad suggestions for the parents when giving these children directives.

1. State the directive simply as possible.
2. Be specific (step by step).
3. Make sure they have eye contact when you talk with them.
4. Reduce external stimuli, if possible.
5. Ask child to repeat directions to ensure his understanding.
6. Don't give too many directions at one time.
7. Be prepared to repeat the directions more than once (and slowly).
8. Keep things as organized as possible (you may have to have lists and charts all over the house).
9. Recognize that this may never go away. In other words, plan on having to do this for a number of years.
10. Recognize that they may often misunderstand what you say.

a. PUNISHMENT & REWARDS

Most parents use a "time out" technique. When using this with ADD children, you must remember that they usually have a poor concept of time. Therefore, 5 minutes may be as effective as 30 minutes. It is usually difficult for the child to stand in a corner or sit in a chair for 30 minutes. They may get into trouble several times before the time has expired. By the end of the time out, they may have forgotten why the punishment was given. A kitchen timer is a good way of structuring these time out periods.

1. WORK - I personally feel that this is one of the best punishment techniques. For example, when a youngster is told that his punishment is to wash the windows in the kitchen, the amount of time that he is punished is put on his shoulders. Until this job is finished, he is restricted from everything.

What is important here, is not the amount of work he has to do, but the fact that he sees that the amount of time spent on restriction is his responsibility. He can't accuse his parents of keeping him on restriction for 5 or 10 hours, because he has control of how fast his job can be completed.

Small amounts of work are recommended, especially for younger children, because this allows parents the opportunity to give out more than one punishment at a time. If you give the child large jobs, they may feel overwhelmed and never start. You must also note that between the time that they start and finish the first job, they may get into trouble again. Therefore, if you gave them a big job the first time, what do you do now? This is one of the reasons I do not like to use <u>time</u> restriction. If a youngster is grounded for a week, it is highly possible that they will get into trouble again during that week. Therefore, they are grounded again. Soon, the child may be grounded until next year. Since this means that they must stay in the house, now the parent is being punished. ADD children usually get into more trouble than non-ADD children. Consequently, more punishment is going to be given to these children. This means that more options have to be available in order to address the large number of misbehaviors.

2. REWARD SYSTEM - This is the technique in which chips, tokens, money, stars, or some other "currency" is used to give to the child for positive behaviors. This is a method that is often used by professionals. Unfortunately, they some-times get so wrapped up in devising the system, that it becomes too complicated to implement. I suggest keeping it simple and use your own imag-ination. I will give a few suggestions but the parent may have to revise it for their particular situation.

I like to use poker chips. If more than one child is involved, I suggest that you use a different color for each. Having a jar for the child to store the poker chips allows them to see what they have earned. This system can be on an hourly, daily, or weekly basis. Actually, the sooner the child receives a reward for their behavior, the better.

Here is how the system works.
. Find the target behavior. (The behavior or task that they are not accomplishing.)

- Reward them with a chip when they do this task better than they have before. In other words, we are trying to get them to improve upon their present behavior. This means we must reward them for gradual improvements even if they do not complete the task the way we want it done. We are planning for the future.
- When handing them a chip, tell them in simple terms what it is for. Do not go into a long explanation because they are unlikely to remember all of it.
- At the end of the week, you allow the child to "cash in" the chips. This could be in the form of money, toys, visits, or whatever you feel the child enjoys. The weight or a- mount of each chip is up to you. Each chip may be worth a penny, nickel, or whatever.

Let me give you an example. If a child has to be told 10 times before she complies, this may be the target behavior. You now reward the child with a chip when you only have to tell them 9 times. After awhile, you wait until they only have to be told 8 times, then 7 times, etc. You want the child to recognize that the parent is paying attention to their "good" behavior. The theory behind this is that when a behavior is rewarded (reinforced) this behavior is more likely to recur. Remember this is the theory, but it doesn't always work. It may take awhile before you see results. I have found that one technique may work for a few weeks or months and then lose it's effectiveness. This means that you may have to alternate between 2 or more systems.

b. SCHOOL RELATED PROBLEMS

Most ADD children have some kind of trouble at school. This is usually related to their distractibility and short attention span. I will now list techniques that may be used by teachers.

1. SUGGESTIONS FOR TEACHERS

- Use heavy outlining on paper in order for the child to distinguish between what is important.
- Allow a child to run errands or stand by desk to give them a "break".
- Sometimes a study booth reduces external stimuli.
- Head phones may have to be used if they have "super hearing".
- Assignments should be short and simple.
- Assignments should be broken into small parts to be completed before receiving another.
- Arrange seating for maximum attention. This may require seating at front of room.
- Follow up after child begins a task.
- Alternate work done at desk with other activities to allow for movement.
- Allow the child a few sample trials of a new task for them to gain familiarity.
- Try to keep child's desk tops uncluttered.
- When correcting their papers, be specific as to what they missed and why.
- Try to avoid correcting the child in an embarrassing manner. Remember, they may not be sensitive to the feelings of others, but they are sensitive to their own.

2. SUGGESTIONS FOR PARENTS

- A daily assignment sheet may be needed to insure that the child does her homework.
- A daily or weekly "report card" may be necessary to follow her progress. These children

usually overestimate their performance and are shocked when they receive a failing grade.
. Do not make them study immediately after school. Allow them a winding down period before starting the homework.
. Provide a quiet and secluded work area.
. Have patience when explaining difficult concepts to the child.
. Help child organize his approach to the homework. Also, have a certain place to keep all books and materials so as to avoid having to search the house the next morning.

C
OTHER TREATMENT METHODS

1. ALLERGIES.
Research has discovered that most of these children have allergies and asthma. This is one area in which there is much controversy. Many believe that if this is treated, the symptoms previously stated, will disappear. Some research indicates that treating allergies does indeed help. The biggest abundance of research indicates that treating allergies does not help to the extent that medication does.

2. REDUCE SUGAR INTAKE.
This is recommeded for all children. It is evident that sugar does increase the activity level of many children. However, ADD is a neurological problem and the removal of sugar does not solve the problem. Again, medication has been found to be much more effective than reducing intake of sugar.

3. NUTRITION/VITAMINS.
Research is contradictory in this area. I personally feel that this area may eventually provide

an alternative treatment that will be effective. There are a lot of claims about the effective treatment of ADD with vitamins and mineral supplements. At this point in time, I would have a difficult time in suggesting this approach over that of medication. The major reason is that I know how a child's life can be affected if he isn't treated early. If we try to use a method that has not been proven to be effective, we are taking a chance on this child's future. Therefore, I would suggest waiting until more substantial studies have been done on the use of vitamins, minerals, and nutrition.

4.   CANDIDAS ALBICANS.
    I must mention this yeast connected illness. It is a relatively new discovery among allergists. There are very few clinics in the country which deal with this problem. The symptoms of this illness are very similar to that of ADD. The only difference is that other physical problems may occur if this illness is present. The basic problem centers around the weakening of the immune system through the exposure to foods, environmental toxins, and some types of medicine. The treatment of candidas albicans involves a change of diet, vitamins, and medication. There have been some rather astonishing results, especially with adults, who have had some problems that resemble ADD. Anyway, I felt this discovery was worth mentioning and I feel that it will become more well known as the years go by.

CHAPTER IX

IMPROVEMENTS SEEN
AFTER
MEDICATION

I must first state that all children respond differently to medication. Just as they exhibit different traits of ADD, they exhibit different responses when treated with medication.

ACADEMIC/LEARNING

Some children make an almost miraculous turnaround. Their grades go from F's to A's. This is primarily due to their increased ability to concentrate and complete a task. They are now able to sit and do their homework without getting up every three minutes. They are also more likely to comprehend what they are studying. They no longer have to push themselves as hard in order to understand what is being taught.

Medication will not cure a learning disability. However, a child who has ADD and a learning disability can be helped through the use of medication. The medication may improve the child's ability to concentrate and retain the information being taught. Consequently, their learning disability can be helped, indirectly, through the increased ability to concentrate.

Many children appear to become more organized in their approach to school. They can keep things orderly and are more likely than before to remember their school work. Their handwriting and work in general may become neater.

They are less likely to become distracted by other students and consequently become more attentive to what is being taught. Because he is now more attentive, the teacher is more likely to respond more positively toward him. He can now follow directions without having to get out of his seat every 3 or 4 minutes to ask the teacher a question.

BEHAVIOR

Because the medication appears to allow the child to think before he acts, his behavior is likely to be less impulsive and unpredictable. Now, he is less likely to butt into games or activities without being invited.

He may now be able to work for long term goals rather than seeking immediate satisfaction. In other words, the parents may be able to use a reward system in which they reward him at the end of the week rather than daily.

Now the child may be able to follow through on tasks. He can retain his concentration long enough to complete a directive. He becomes more trustworthy.

He is less likely to interrupt conversations between peers or adults. He is more able to wait his turn to speak. Waiting in lines, such as at the cafeteria or grocery store, becomes easier.

He may have more patience. He may only have to be told to do something 2 or 3 times instead of 6 or 7.

He may become more careful in his play. He becomes less accident prone. In other words, he may no longer seek exciting and dangerous things to do. The medication seems to lower the pain tolerance to within the average range. Consequently, he can now feel things that he couldn't previously. He can also see the possible danger signals of an activity. He may now remember that his parents told him not to engage in a particular activity, and refrain from doing so.

He may become more responsible with money. He may be able to save his money for a particular item without giving in to temptation of spending it impulsively.

His understanding of morality may become more pronounced. His taking of items without paying for them may decrease. He is now more able to understand the explanations of his parents, concerning stealing.

When dealing with a difficult task, he is less likely to become frustrated and have a temper tantrum.

EMOTIONAL

When considering the aforementioned improvements in learning and behavior, it should be easy to decipher some of the emotional benefits of taking medication. Because he has controlled some of his behavior, his relationships may become more positive. He may not be rejected by his peers, which improves his feelings of self-worth. Adults may not be as negative with him. With parents, he may experience more positive inter-actions than ever before. He may no longer feel left out of the family unit.

Improvement in school and lessened negative behaviors will also result in a more enhanced self-image. He may no longer feel dumb. Teachers may no longer have to punish him as much.

The improvements seen on medication are not evident in every child. Some may show drama-tic improvement, some may show moderate im-provement. Of course, there are those children who will show no improvement. Research shows that about 20% of these children will not respond to medication.

CHAPTER X

DEALING WITH OTHER AGENCIES

In this chapter I will cover problems that I have run into after a child has been diagnosed as ADD. As mentioned earlier, diagnosing ADD is difficult and sometimes talking the parents into treating the child with medication is also difficult. At this point it may appear that the hardest part is over. Unfortunately, this is not true. When you have to deal with people in other agencies, your patience will be tested to the limit. Therefore, I am including this chapter in order to inform you that diagnosing and treating the child is only the first step.

SCHOOL SYSTEMS

Most children with ADD have learning problems of some kind. Behavior problems are also common. Consequently, the school system and the parents will get to know each other well. Sometimes this relationship is rocky. The parents may blame the teachers and other personnel for the child's problems. The teachers may, in turn, blame the parents for the child's problem.

Since most of these children have some type of learning problem or behavior problem, special meetings are usually held between the parents and school personnel. This meeting may include the school counselor, diagnostician, a resource teacher, and possibly the principal, or vice-principal. The meetings are conducted in order to develop an educational plan for this child. Before this meeting can be conducted, testing must be done on the child. These tests will determine the areas in which the child may need help, or determine whether or not the child qualifies for any special educational placement. The unfortunate thing about the testing, is that it is inadequate for determining the presence of ADD. One reason for this is that when a child is tested, he is usually in a quiet room with an adult. In such a setting the child is able to concentrate and perform adequately. This usually means that the child may score high enough on the tests that he will not qualify for special help. Therefore, he must remain where he is. Ironically, when he is placed back in the classroom with twenty other children, he is not able to concentrate and pay attention as well as he did in the testing session. Hence, he may end up failing in these classes.

This is the problem I run into in many of these meetings. The child has obtained a high score that does not qualify him for special help even though he may be failing. The school personnel are likely to state that there's nothing they can do for him because of his scores. This is not true. Parents are usually unaware of their rights at these meetings and usually go along with the suggestions of the school personnel. If a parent does question what the committee has decided, they are sometimes treated in a rude manner. This is because they do not like their decisions to be challenged. This is not unusual for any human being. None of us like our integrity challenged. This is how most committee members interpret a parent's questions. At this point in time, the meeting may become rather unfriendly.

I personally feel that a child with ADD should be given special help even though the testing scores do not indicate this. To obtain this help, it may require a more aggressive and confrontational approach to the committee members. I personally do not like to argue, but I have discovered that if you are going to help out this child you may have to become rather stern. If the parent does this without a therapist present, the committee members are likely to conclude that the child's problems are a result of having to put up with this pushy parent. Some parents have been blatantly told that they are less than adequate as parents. Needless to say, many parents have broken down into tears at these meetings. As you know, this usually renders someone helpless in defending themselves in an argument.

My major point is that you must prepare yourself for the possibility of a confrontation with these members. It is best to remain cool and speak on an intellectual level to avoid the members becoming defensive. It is also important to take a representative with you. You may be told that you are not allowed to have any outside individuals attend this meeting. This is merely an attempt to intimidate you and is also a violation of federal regulations. You are allowed to choose anyone to attend these meetings on your behalf.

Some of my clients have been told by school personnel, that I would not be allowed to attend a meeting. The reason that they didn't want me to come was because they know that I understand what they can and can't do for a child. The parent is not aware of the options and may give in to what the school officials recommend, even if it isn't what is best for the child.

I will now give you a list of reasons why it is important that you ask for this official meeting:

1. First of all, it may be good to explain to the committee members that your child has ADD. They may not always welcome this news, especially if your child has been tested by the school system over a number of years and they have overlooked this diagnosis. They may question whether or not this is the true problem.

2. Just because your child has been placed on medication, he will not automatically begin learning at a faster rate. There is no way that he can recuperate the knowledge that he has not gained from being inattentive in class over the past few years. Being on the medicine will allow him to learn more effectively, but it will not effect his past. Therefore, it will be necessary to place him in easier classes for 1/2 year or so in order to allow him to catch up.

3. If placing him in easier classes is not possible, it may be necessary to lower his mastery level. In other words, if 70% is usually considered passing, the committee has the right to lower the mastery level. This means that the child only has to make a 60% to pass.

4. If your child failed or almost failed the past year, you may request that he go ahead into the next grade anyway. Many people disagree with this procedure. I have found that when a child is on medication, there is a better chance that they can perform adequately with their school work. The argument the school personnel may give is that they feel the child will either mature or buckle down and study next year. In other words they are indirectly stating that they do not believe that the child has a physiological problem and that the reason they failed was due to their not putting forth effort. Another reason for requesting advancement into the next grade is because his failure was not necessarily his fault. If he has ADD, and has been overlooked for a number of years, he has probably been placed in the wrong classes. My contention is, that the school system would make special arrangements for a child who failed physical education if a physiological problem was discovered. Most people would agree that a child should not be held responsible for having a physical problem. This is the case with ADD children. This is a physical problem that has been overlooked. Failing them because of this is not proper.

5. I have found that when a child is on medication, it appears to be most effective in the morning hours. Therefore, I suggest that the child's most difficult subject be scheduled for the morning, if that is possible. Their attention span and their ability to concentrate is at a higher level at this time.

If you have trouble at this meeting and you feel that the committee members are not doing their best for your child, you have other alternatives. The following is the procedure you should use if you feel a better plan could be developed for your child:

..The first step begins at the end of this special meeting. At the end of the meeting, a piece of paper is passed around for the committee members to sign that they agree or disagree with the decision. You have the right to mark disagree and write the reasons for this disagreement. You can make this as long as you want and attach as many sheets as you desire. It is extremely important to check the disagree column on this piece of paper. If you sign agree, then you have basically said that you agree with everything. You then have no rights to complain.

..After this meeting you may contact the principal, if he wasn't at the meeting, and tell him what you would like. If he can do nothing, then you go on to the next step.

..You now have the right to send a letter to the State Commissioner of Education and request a mediator. This step-by-step procedure is in a pamphlet that is given to the parents of children who go to these special meetings. If you do not have one, request it from the counselor. Do not let the numerous pages and headings frighten you. This procedure is very simple and takes very little time. After the Commissioner of Education receives your letter, you will be contacted by someone from that office. Within two weeks you will have a meeting with somebody from their office, as well as someone from the local school system. At this meeting, you go through the same procedure we previously mentioned. The difference is, that you now have an impartial third party who is probably less defensive or emotionally involved.

..If this mediation process does not provide what you would like, request a hearing. This is more like a legal meeting. The education agency will provide an attorney for their side and will suggest that you bring one. This is not necessary, you may bring a therapist who is familiar with this disorder if you would like or you can present your case alone.

..If you do not get satisfaction from this meeting, you have another alternative. You may file suit against the school system. I hate to mention this because it sounds like I'm a radical who is out to get the school. This is not the case. We must remember that the purpose of these meetings are to obtain what is best for the child. As stated throughout this book, the consequences of a child not getting the proper treatment can be devastating. Therefore, I feel that it is important to go to any length to do what is best for the child.

DEPARTMENT OF HUMAN SERVICES

Dealing with case workers is sometimes difficult. You must remember that they have very little, if any, background knowledge of ADD. What background knowledge they may have is incomplete and very narrow. You must remember that their training is primarily in the area of family and they are, therefore, geared towards explaining things in terms of family dynamics.

This means that if a child is disruptive at home or is disciplined more than most children, the first thing a case worker will do is assess the parents. Their assumption is that the parents are the primary cause of a child's behavior. They are likely to overlook a physiological explanation for this behavior.

As mentioned earlier, most of the families of these children are disorganized. Consequently, the case worker will witness this disorganization and jump to conclusions. If a child has been reported to the department for being abused, the parents may be forced into counseling. I have discovered that a number of parents who come for counseling, accused of child abuse, state that their child is difficult to handle, doesn't pay attention, and usually has trouble in school. In other words, a lot of these parents have children who have ADD. If you remember, one of the characteristics of these children is that they sometimes have a high tolerance for pain. This means that spankings are not effective in controlling the child's behavior. Unfortunately, parents become frustrated and angry and may spank the child harder than usual in order for them to feel the pain. When this is done, either marks or broken skin may result. If this is seen by someone, the parent may be turned in for child abuse.

When a case worker becomes involved in the family, one of the first things they suggest is that the parent no longer spank the child. This is not only a suggestion, it is backed by law. The parents are likely to become even more frustrated, because no other form of discipline is effective. The parents may be sent for counseling, and the therapist is not likely to consider the child as having a problem. Because the parents are defensive, angry, and frustrated, the therapist may conclude that this is the major problem. He will then start to work on the parents and suggest child rearing techniques and continue this therapy for months. This will be done while the major problem is being overlooked.

I have worked with numerous parents who have been in the above situation. I have talked with the case workers and have told them that the child needs to be treated with medication. As soon as a case worker hears medication, they automatically assume the reason we want to pre-scribe it is so the child will be drugged up and the parents won't have to deal with the child's behavior. They do not understand that the medication is for the child's benefit. Caseworkers usually feel that if the parents would just get their act together, their children's problems would disappear.

Another problem that may be encountered with case workers is their age. You must remember that many case workers have not been out of college very long. This means they may be in their mid-twentys. They may or may not be mar-ried. If they are married, their children will be very young. This means that they not only lack experience with ADD children, they usually lack experience with the average child. Consequently, most of their theories about children are based on book knowledge and idealism. This makes it difficult for them to understand ADD and the effect these children will have upon the family's situation.

JUVENILE PROBATION DEPARTMENTS

The primary contact that professionals have with Juvenile Probation Offices is when testing is requested. Not every child who goes through the probation office receives testing. Those youngsters who may be sent to a child care facility must receive testing before they can be accepted. It is here that a lot of ADD youngsters are misdiagnosed and consequently referred for the wrong treatment. (This is paid for by the taxpayers.)

I am often accused of over-diagnosing ADD. I find that the major reason that I am accused of this is because other professionals hardly diagnose it. Even though it is more common in children than any diagnosis or disorder, other clinicians rarely diagnose it.

For example, a common diagnostic category many professionals use is that of conduct disorder. It is rather easily defined: a conduct disorder is a person or child who exhibits negative behaviors and becomes involved in illegal activities. This diagnosis is very common among kids who are handled by the juvenile justice system. When these kids come to the attention of a juvenile probation office, they are sometimes referred for testing.

Since the child is referred for testing by a juvenile probation office, the professional doing the testing is aware that the child must be in trouble because of his conduct. As you might guess, this narrows down the diagnostic categories in which this child may fit. At this point, I feel that many professionals diagnose the child as having conduct disorder. This is done before the child is tested. In other words, the professional

reverses the normal procedure. Instead of testing
the child in order to develop a diagnosis, a diagnosis is developed before testing has taken place.
Of course the professional will not admit to that,
but it is obvious, due to the large number of
children diagnosed as conduct disorders.

Consequently, the majority of kids seen by
a juvenile probation office are diagnosed as conduct
disorders. At this point I must explain from where
these diagnostic names of conduct disorder and
ADD come.

There is a book called The DSM III that is
put out by the American Psychiatric Association.
It is considered the authority in the United States
for mental disorders. DSM III stands for Diagnostic
and Statistical Manual. All professionals in the
United States use this book when diagnosing anyone.
I should say, that every professional in the United
States should use this book when diagnosing someone. I have found that many professionals go by
their "gut" reaction and ignore the research in
the DSM III.

In the DSM III, ADD is listed and it tells
you how to diagnose it. It also tells you what
to look for in order to avoid misdiagnosing it.
Conduct disorder is listed in the DSM III as well.
The characteristics common to conduct disorders
are listed in order to allow for a proper diagnosis.
This is also done in order to avoid misdiagnosing
conduct disorder.

I have worked and tested for many probation
offices and have found that a large number of
kids who get into trouble have ADD. Research
also indicates this fact. Consequently, when I

do testing on a child from the probation office, they sometimes have the diagnosis of ADD and conduct disorder. When the probation office sees the diagnosis over and over again, they eventually assume that I know how to diagnose nothing but ADD. Especially when they see that other professionals don't include ADD as a diagnosis. What really disturbs them is that my recommendation is to start the child on medication. The reason for this, of course, is obvious. Medication is the only treatment effective for ADD. To support my claims I usually get the DSM III and turn to conduct disorders. Within the characteristics of conduct disorders it is clearly stated on three separate occasions that Attention Deficit Disorder is common among children with conduct disorders. In fact, ADD is one of the major reasons a child becomes a behavior problem.

Even with this information so blatantly written in the DSM III, I am amazed at how many professionals in the United States do not diagnose conduct disorders along with ADD. What this suggests is, that there are thousands of kids in the United States that are being misdiagnosed and consequently, mistreated. The treatment for ADD is different than the treatment for conduct disorder.

ADD is more common than conduct disorders. Yet I am sure that many of you who are reading about this today are not aware of ADD. You are probably more aware of conduct disorders.

If every juvenile probation office in the United States was examined thoroughly, I would venture to guess that over 95% of the children have been diagnosed as conduct disorders. Although ADD is very common and a cause of youngsters having conduct disorders, I would also venture to guess that less than 5% of these kids would even have ADD mentioned as a possible problem.

Most probation departments have been working with a select group of professionals for years. Since these professionals don't diagnose these kids as having ADD, the department will question the judgement of someone who disagrees with them. Since these professionals have no motivation to become more aware of ADD, they will continue misdiagnosing these kids and sending them for treatment that will prove ineffective. In essence, they will continue to waste the taxpayers money on improper treatment techniques. More importantly, they will continue ruining kids lives by overlooking their main problems.

ADOPTION AGENCIES

The reason I'm mentioning adoption agencies is due to several reasons. First of all, research indicates that adopted children are 4 times more likely to have ADD than non-adopted children. Remember, ADD is hereditary. This means that one of the parents of the adopted child probably has ADD.

There is no research that supports the following statements I will make. When we consider the characteristics of a person with ADD, we may understand why so many adopted children have this disorder. If one of the parents has ADD, they are prone to be impulsive, thrill seeking, and not consider the consequences of their actions. When this person reaches the teen years, sexual urges arise. Due to their lack of impulse control, they are more likely to act on these urges. Due to their inability to consider the consequences of their actions, it is unlikely that they will use a form of contraception. Because these individuals are young and irresponsible, it is unlikely that they are able to care for a child. Consequently, if they become pregnant they must give the child up for adoption. (Most children given up for adoption are born to young parents.)

Again, there is no research that supports my theory as to why the natural parents of ADD children must give up their children for adoption. Research does indicate that adopted children are 4 times more likely to have ADD than non-adoptive children. This much is a fact!

Another reason I am mentioning adoption agencies is because of their apparent lack of knowledge regarding the large number of adopted children who have ADD. For example, I wrote to an adoption agency telling them about a young pregnant girl who was coming to them to give up her child for adoption. This girl was diagnosed as having ADD. Therefore, I told them that there is a high probability that her child will have ADD, especially if it is a boy. I went on to say that the adoptive parents should be made aware of this fact because they may start having problems with the child when they are 6 or 7 years of age. I also quoted research which noted that adoptive children need counseling intervention more often than non-adopted children. I felt that the major reason that these children were sent for counseling was due to the fact that they had ADD. In essence, I challenged the contemporary theory of why adopted children seek counseling. The view held by most people is that adopted children need counseling in order to resolve their feelings of abandonment or their desire to find their "roots". I'm sure that this happens, at times. But, I feel that the major reason that most adopted children are sent for counseling is due to the symptoms of ADD. Since these children are very likely to have ADD, they may have behavioral or learning problems at an early age. Because the parents are aware of the "theory" of adopted children, they may assume that this is why their child is having problems. When others discover that the child is adopted, they may assume the same "theory". Consequently, the child may be referred for counseling in order for them to resolve these feelings. Unfortunately, this is the wrong treatment and little progress will be made in the area of behavior or learning. In fact, I feel that counseling these young children about being adopted inserts ideas about being adopted that they would never have thought about otherwise. This could lead to the child becoming obsessed with their natural parents. Remember, ADD children are prone to exaggerate what they hear. They are also prone to more intense feelings. Therefore, they may become extremely emotionally involved in this topic. Although it may not have been a problem before, it could become one.

My major point, is that adopted children are very likely to have ADD. This means that they will have the problems commonly associated with ADD (i.e., behavior, learning). Therefore, when an adopted child exhibits problems, it is more likely to be due to the ADD rather than the fact that they are adopted.

CHILDREN'S HOMES

Most of the children at childrens' homes are usually referred through a juvenile probation department. As previously mentioned, most of these youngsters are usually diagnosed as conduct disorders. Although ADD is often the cause of this conduct disorder, it usually goes undiagnosed. Consequently, the treatment program that this facility may implement will be directed at the conduct disorder and not ADD. Again, the major problem is not being treated.

Although these children may have obvious learning problems and are enrolled in a resource class, the facility will still focus treatment on the conduct disorder and not ADD. These youngsters may show improvement over a few months. When they are put back in the home environment, they are likely to resume their old behavior patterns.

If a child is put in a psychiatric hospital, they may be placed on medication. The medication may help this ADD child. Improvement may be dramatic. Unfortunately, when they are released from the hospital, the parents are not told the importance of the medication. Consequently, the parent may stop getting the prescription filled and the child's behavior and learning problems may reappear.

If the parent is given a detailed account of the benefits of the medication, I feel that they would be more inclined to insist that the child take it.

There are numerous children in the hospitals who have ADD but are not diagnosed. Consequently, they are receiving the wrong treatment at a cost of about $7,000.00 per month. Insurance companies pay the largest portion of these fees. Champus, the military insurance company, pays 80% of this fee. This is money that you, the taxpayer, are furnishing for a child to be mistreated. In other words, we are paying millions of dollars every year for children in psychiatric facilities to receive the wrong treatment.

(Note: I have described some of the difficult problems with which you may encounter in dealing with various agencies. Not all agencies make things difficult. Some are cooperative. What matters is the type of person with which you're dealing. Needless to say, I have run into some difficult people and I felt that I should warn the reader of the problems that could arise.)

CHAPTER XI

REASON ADD MAY BE OVERLOOKED

Professionals lack of knowledge..........................

Most professionals have heard of ADD, but their knowledge is incomplete. Therefore, if a child's symptoms do not fit into their realm of knowledge, the child will not be diagnosed as ADD.

Conscientious Parents.......................

Parents who have ADD children may be extremely conscientious and spend a great deal of time working with the child. They may spend so much time helping them with homework or putting forth extraordinary efforts to organize the child, that no one may notice the child having a severe problem. In essence, the parent has "masked" the ADD through hard work.

Extremely High Intelligence................

If a child is extremely intelligent, she may be able to go through the first few years of school making adequate grades. This kind of child may eventually become "burned out" emotionally, due to the frustrations of pushing themselves to concentrate.

ADD Children Without Hyperactivity...............

Since these children are usually quiet and perhaps passive, teachers may not recognize that they have a problem. They may assume the child is having problems at home instead of the presence of ADD.

Child is a Teenager...................

Most professionals come in contact with ADD children in the 1st to 4th grades. If a child is a teenager, they assume that the youngsters couldn't have ADD because she would have been discovered at an earlier age.

Behavioral Problem..................

If a child is resistant and non-compliant, most people assume that the child chooses this behavior. They may not consider the child having ADD. Lack of impulse control is a common problem with these youngsters. They act before they think.

Sibling With ADD......................

If a sibling has ADD and exhibits extremely negative behaviors, the other child may appear to be perfect in comparison. Therefore, if this child has ADD but not to the severe degree of the sibling, they may go overlooked for years.

Family Problems......................

If the parents are having marital problems, this may be seen as the reason the child is having behavioral or academic problems. Most people do not realize that more than one problem may exist in a child's life. Most professionals focus on the environmental circumstances in the child's life and ignore the possibility of ADD being a problem.

Other Problems in Child's Life..................

When other events have occurred in a child's life (i.e., divorce, abuse, etc.) ADD is unlikely to be seen as a problem. These other areas are more readily observed. Hence, the focus of treatment.

Child is Black or Other Minority..................

I have found that most of white America still has a stereotyped view of minorities, especially blacks. When a black child exhibits the symptoms of having ADD (i.e., resistant behavior, bossiness, difficulty in learning) it is likely to be seen as cultural. In other words, if a black child is having trouble in school, teachers or other professionals may subconsciously accept this as a common trait among blacks and not a symptom of the child having ADD. I have witnessed several black youngsters who had been overlooked but exhibited obvious traits of ADD. If a white child had exhibited the same traits, the chances are, that they would have been referred for help at an earlier age.

CHAPTER XII

QUESTIONS AND ANSWERS

Q. 1. How can I tell if my child's behavior is out of the ordinary or just a normal type of behavior?

A. Many people feel that the descriptions given about ADD children are common to every child they have ever seen. I agree that every child exhibits the behaviors that I have described. The difference between the average child and the ADD child is one of degree. For example: Every child misbehaves but children with ADD will usually misbehave more than others. Every child has trouble learning at some point. However, children with ADD usually have more trouble learning than others. To answer your question more directly, I would suggest that you use the evaluation methods which are stated in an earlier chapter. These are arranged in such a manner so as to avoid diagnosing a child who doesn't have ADD. You must remember that every child is different. A common misconception is that if you have seen one ADD child you've seen them all. This is not true. One child may be extremely active, while another child may be withdrawn. One child may have learning problems and another may not demonstrate learning problems until the seventh or eighth grade. Again, using the evaluation method should help you distinguish the difference between ordinary behavior and that of ADD children.

Q. 2. Is the medication they take addictive?

A.   No. The children do not end up craving this medication. Research indicates that if a child with ADD takes medication at an early age it reduces the chances that he will abuse drugs in the later years.

Q. 3. I have been to a doctor on several occasions questioning whether or not my child had ADD. My physician, whom we trust and love, says that he doesn't feel the child has ADD and will not prescribe medication. What should I do?

A.   I would suggest that if you feel that your child has ADD, you show this evidence to your doctor. You may have to challenge him and believe me, this may mean that your relationship will deteriorate. I have discovered that most people do not like to be second-guessed. Many people do not question a physician's authority and therefore they do as he requests. This is the easy way out. You must remember that your primary motive for seeking treatment is for your child's benefit. Therefore, a choice may have to be made between the friendship of your physician and the future of your child. If your physician does not respond to the information you have given him based on what you have learned in this book and through other articles, I would suggest that you go seek another physician or therapist. You should question their ability to diagnose ADD. You must remember also that if you ask a professional whether or not they are familiar with ADD, it is likely that they will say yes. Almost all professionals have heard of ADD. The unfortunate thing is that their knowledge of this disorder is incomplete. This may result in them misdiagnosing the disorder because the child does not fit into the category that they have designated as ADD. To challenge a professional further, I suggest that you take this book, along with the DSM III (Diagnostic and Statistical Manual of the American Psychiatric Association). Most therapists have the DSM III. I would suggest that you have them turn to the pages relating to Attention Deficit Disorder. Ask them to go over the criteria with you and the two of you will determine whether or not your child fits into this category. This may be the best way to challenge their knowledge.

Q. 4. I am an adult and feel that I have had this disorder when I was younger. Is there anything I can do now to help this problem?

A.   Yes, there is treatment for adults. I have successfully treated several adults who have had a history of alcohol and drug abuse. I have treated adults who have been diagnosed as having other mental problems. I have treated adults who have been placed in mental institutions but received little help. It is more difficult to diagnose an adult than it is a child. This is because numerous other problems may have arisen over the years. Now it will be difficult to distinguish between what is due to the disorder and what is due to other factors. I would suggest that you go to your medical doctor with the information in this book. I would tell him that you felt as if you had this disorder when you were younger and still suffer from the side effects. Then show him the part of the book in which the treatment for adults is given. Most doctors will recognize that Tofranil is a relatively safe medication and will not be too fearful of prescribing it.

Q. 5. My child refuses to take the medication. What can I do?

A.   If the child has a difficult time swallowing pills, I would suggest that you ask your doctor to give you this medication in the liquid form or a chewable tablet. You probably had to develop some method of giving other medication to your child, therefore it may be necessary to try the same technique. If, however, the major problem is the child doesn't want to take the medication because of the way it makes him feel, the dosage level may need to be examined. The dosage may be too high and you may have to reduce it for a time until the child's body becomes used to it. If the child is obstinate and refuses to take the medication, you may have to resort to discipline in order for him to take it.

Q. 6. Teachers at school complain that they have problems with my son. The strange thing is, that I don't have the same problems at home. I think it may be the teacher's fault and not the child's. What do you think?

A. Remember, children with ADD do not exhibit negative behaviors in all situations. They may do well at home but do poorly at school or vice versa. Therefore, I would be inclined to listen to what the teacher says. This may indicate that your child needs medication. This is not the only manner in which ADD is diagnosed but it is important to listen to what the teachers say. I will agree that many times, teachers create some of the problems with the children but that still doesn't mean that your child doesn't have a problem.

Q. 7. My child is ten years old and is on Ritalin but it makes him worse instead of better. What should we do?

A. Of all medications used for children, Ritalin has some of the most detrimental side effects. I would suggest that you ask your physician to try the child on Cylert. When you say that the medicine makes him worse instead of better, I

would have to ask about which time of
day he seems worse, mornings or evenings?
Many times, the side effect of this medication is that the child may become a little
more hyper as it wears off in the evenings.
You must remember that when children
go through puberty, the type of medication
must be changed. If not, Ritalin or other
stimulants, may make them worse. Although your son is only ten years old
it may be a good idea to have a physician examine him to determine whether
or not he may be going through puberty
at an early age. I have seen some kids
who have gone through puberty at ten
or eleven.

Q. 8.   My husband absolutely refuses to put
our child on medication. He has been
diagnosed as ADD. How should we approach
him? What can we do?

A.   Someone who is familiar with this disorder
needs to talk with you and your husband.
I have found many parents very negative
about the idea of medicine for their child
until I have pointed out the possible results
of the child not taking the medication.
Research indicates that children who
were not treated at an early age have
a higher probability of becoming alcohol
or drug abusers in the teenage and adult
years. Research also indicates that people
not treated are more prone to illegal
activities. I am not saying that it is definitely the case that your child will become involved with the law or become
a drug abuser if he doesn't take the med-

icine. What I am saying is that this is a physiological problem, (chemical imbalance) and it needs to be treated properly. Ask your husband if he would refuse giving a crippled child a wheelchair to ride in. Would he suggest that someone with high blood pressure not take medication? Of course not. This is the case with your child. If he has ADD, this is a physiological problem that needs to be treated with medication. If it is not treated properly you are allowing your child to suffer with a disorder that could be easily treated. What I would suggest is ask your husband if he would be willing to try the medication for two months. If, within two months an improvement is not noticed, then you can take the child off the medication. I have found that most parents do this for a short time. Once they see the positive outcome, they are more likely to believe that medication is needed.

Q. 9. I have two children that are almost opposite in their personalities but seem to have some problems that are similar. Is it possible that both could have ADD but show different signs?

A. Yes, it is possible that more than one child in a family can have this disorder. Remember, this disorder is hereditary and is very likely to occur in boys rather than girls. Therefore, if you have two boys there is a high probability that both could have the disorder. Sometimes the child who has the disorder may cause some problems within the family. This

may result in the other child appearing
to have problems when in reality they
are only reacting to the ADD child's
behavior. Younger children have a tendency
to model after the older sibling. Consequently, they could be modeling the older
child's behavior. Also, not all ADD children
exhibit the same characteristics. For
example: one child's major problems could
be in the area of learning and another
child's major problems could be in having
temper outbursts. In other words, they
may have problems that are dissimilar.
It would take a good diagnostic evaluation
to determine whether or not both have
the disorder. I have discovered that other
professionals have questioned the chances
of two children in the same family having
this disorder. Again, what they don't
understand is, that it is more likely to
occur in the siblings of ADD children.
The major problem you may run into is
when both children are placed on medication. To others, this will appear as if
all you want to do is dope up your children
so they are easier to handle. You will
have to put up with this kind of criticism
from all types of people.

Q. 10. I disagree with putting children on medication for this disorder. I feel that these
children are screaming for love and affection. I feel that most of their behavior
is a striving for attention.

A.   I agree with your statements about these
children seeking love and affection and
that their acting out behavior is for atten-

tion. But, you must remember that if a child has ADD, they have a physiological problem. It is a chemical imbalance that can only be treated successfully through the use of medication. Often, these children actually do seek more affection and attention than most children. They over-react to most situations. This means that they are also prone to overreaction when seeking attention and approval. The more you give, the more they want. No matter how much love and affection you give an ADD child, this chemical imbalance will not be "cured". People usually observe the parent being rather harsh on these children and they are prone to say something like...."If the parent would show more kindness and love for the child, he would behave." You must remember that the parents have spent several years coping with this child's misbehaviors. They have learned what works and what doesn't work. When you observe their response to these children, they are responding in a manner which they have found to be effective. Therefore, I would suggest that you hold off your judgment until you have lived with these children three or four months. The parents have heard these comments many times. Many parents have drifted into depression and self-doubt because they have a tendency to blame themselves. The parents or no one else should be blamed for this disorder. It is hereditary. Just as we have no control over a child's hair color, we have no control over whether or not he will inherit ADD.   '

Q. 11. ADD sort of sounds like schizophrenia.
        Could it be schizophrenia instead?

A.   You are correct. However, in the DSM
        III (the authority on mental disorders
        in the United States) it is stated that
        before you diagnose a child as ADD you
        rule out other possible disorders. Schizo-
        phrenia is one disorder that must be ruled
        out. I will not go into the differences
        between schizophrenia and ADD but the
        differences are obvious. You must re-
        member that schizophrenia is very rare
        in children and ADD is very common.
        So, from the beginning the odds are with
        ADD. Therefore, before diagnosing schizo-
        phrenia or ADD, the criteria in the DSM
        III should be examined carefully to deter-
        mine which diagnosis is more appropriate.

Q. 12. I am afraid to put my child on medica-
        tion. What other alternatives are there
        other than medicine?

A.   As stated previously there are other alterna-
        tives. However, they have not been proven
        to be as effective as medication. Before
        experimenting with your child's future,
        I would read the section of my book that
        points out what can happen to a child
        if they are not treated at an early age.
        However, I will tell you once again some
        of the other alternatives:
     1. Have allergy testing done. It may prove
        beneficial to treat the child for allergies
        as well as allergy-proof their room. This
        means removing all stuffed animals, carpet-
        ing, putting cheese cloth over air vents
        and plastic over the mattresses.

2. Reducing certain foods and introducing vitamins into their diet. Again this is not proven to be extremely successful but there is some merit to it.

Again, medication has been shown to be the only treatment that is successful. Therefore, I would encourage you to reconsider using the medicine. It could prove to be one of the most important elements of your child's life.

Q. 13. I have seen kids on medication that look like they are drugged. I don't want my child to be this way and I'm afraid this will happen if he gets on medication.

A. Most parents do not realize that when a child first starts medication, his body will not be used to it. Therefore, for the first two or three days he may appear to be drowsy and sluggish. Unfortunately many physicians do not warn the parents before giving the medication. When the parents witness the stupor that the child appears to be in, they are sometimes inclined to discontinue the medication. The truth is, if they had waited a few more days it is very likely that the child's body would have adjusted to the medicine and these side effects would have disappeared. Eventually, you could not tell that the child was on medicine. As pointed out earlier in the book, it is important to know the dosage commonly given to children of a given age. This way, you can tell whether or not your physician may have prescribed too large a dosage. If this occurs, be sure and call your physician and question the dosage level. It is unfortunate, but many parents have taken their child off medication after observing a negative reaction. I have witnessed parents, 8 or 10 years later, who come to me because they are having problems with their child. When I discover that a child was taken off medication at an early age, I explain that if the child had stayed on the medicine it would be unlikely that he would be having the problems that he is today. This doesn't mean that it is too late for treatment, but it does mean that the child has spent several years coping with a problem that could probably have been resolved earlier through the use of medicine.

Q. 14.   Is my child likely to become a drug abuser because he is so used to taking these drugs?

A.   As a matter of fact research shows that children who were treated at an early age were less likely to abuse drugs than the normal population. Note: this means that ADD children who have been treated with medication are more likely to avoid alcohol and drug abuse than non-ADD children. I can't exactly explain this but my theory is that they have become so used to taking medicine that they are tired of it. Another reason may be that when they are taking medication, they are more likely to make better judgments.

Q. 15. If a child is not placed on medication does this definitely mean that he will become an alcohol or drug abuser?

A. No. Just because a child has this disorder and is not treated doesn't mean that they will become alcohol or drug abusers. There are many people who have grown up with ADD and have become successful. They beat the odds. There are more who do not become successful than do. Therefore, I would hope that you do not try to beat the odds.

Q. 16. Does this disorder go away? Will my child have to stay on medication all his life?

A. There are three basic courses of this disorder.
   1. Some symptoms may disappear in puberty (this is usually the excessive activity level.)
   2. All symptoms may remain throughout their life.
   3. All symptoms may disappear before adulthood.

   Unfortunately, no one knows which course a particular child will follow. This has to be done by monitoring the child over time.

   Regarding the medication: some people will need the medication for the rest of their life, some won't. The most important time to be on medication is from 6 - 18 years of age. This is when one's sense of self is developing. Therefore, any problems they may have at this age will have an impact on their self concept.

Q. 17. I have heard that some Doctors suggest that the child be taken off the medication on weekends and in the summer. Do you also suggest this be done?

A.   I do not agree with taking the child off medication during these times. Most physicians feel that the only time the child needs the medication is while he is at school. Because the medication increases their ability to concentrate, they are apt to learn better. The problem with this is that a child also learns things outside of school. In fact, I would say that the things that the child learns outside of school are more important than what they learn in school. For example, a child is more attentive to directives from parents, they listen to and comprehend social situations better, and they are likely to gain more positive feedback when they are on medication. In other words, these youngsters gain a great deal emotionally as well as intellectualy, when they are on the medication in the summer and on weekends. Remember, the medication is for the benefit of the child. Parents and others benefit, but this is not the primary reason the child was placed on medication. If a child behaves and makes better judgements when he is on medication, he will not be disciplined or criticized as often. Obviously, this benefits the child's self-image, while at the same time reducing the parents' stress. I feel that the child should stay on the medication year round.

Q. 18. My child has learning disabilities along with ADD. Will the medication cure the learning disabilities?

A.   No, medication will not "cure" a learning disability. However, the learning disability can be improved upon when the child is on medication. Using simple logic, it is obvious that a child will learn better when his attention span and concentration is at an optimum level. Therefore, when a child is on medication, the remedial help that the child is receiving may be more effective and require less time for the child to comprehend. (Research shows that 60 - 80% of children with learning disabilities also have ADD.)

Q. 19. I have heard that putting a child on medication does not always improve their school performance.

A.   This is true. First of all, I would not use the word "always" when dealing with children with ADD. They are all different and have different problems. They also respond differently to medication. However, based on my experience, I have seen enough children improve their school performance that I am willing to say that the medication will help the child make better grades. If the medication is effective, the child's ability to concentrate and complete tasks is apt to improve. Common sense tells me that the child's school work will im-

prove in direct porportion to his ability
to concentrate and complete his assignments. (Research indicates that medication
does not necessarily improve a child's
grades.) This is one of the few times
that I contradict research findings. However, I have a large number of parents
and youngsters who can testify to the
improvement in school grades after having
been placed on the medication.

Q. 20. My child is having trouble in school but
the principal and teachers feel that the
major problem is his behavior. He doesn't
qualify for special classes but he is failing
in his regular classroom. What can I do?

A.   If you feel the child has ADD, you may
have to press your point. However, it
doesn't matter whether or not the school
officials believe your child has ADD.
What matters is that you want him to
get some help. Continue pressing for
special classes.

What is confusing to the school system
is that when a child is tested to see if
they qualify for special classes, they usually
score too high.

Q. 21. I feel that my child has ADD but the
cost of seeing a professional is beyond
my means. What can I do?

A.   This is an often asked question. In order
to answer this, I usually ask the following
questions: "How many books, jackets,
eye-glasses, toys, bicycles, and other

items has your child lost or destroyed
in the past year?" Children with ADD
do this much more often than the average
child. When treated, they usually become
more organized and can keep up with
things. My point is that it may cost you
more money by not treating the child.
I have only discussed the monetary gains
and losses to this point. When you consider
the emotional factors, it could be extremely expensive to not treat your child.

CHAPTER XIII

CASE REPORTS

CASE REPORT

BILLY

The following was originally printed in the Abilene Reporter News, by Michelle Morris:

Billy seemed to be born in trouble.

From the time he was in an Abilene kindergarten, Billy (names of family members have been changed) was constantly being yelled at, spanked or put in detention for something he had done wrong at school or at home.

He could never finish a project, sit still or remember what the teacher or his parents told him to do. Billy fought with his sister, Lisa, all the time.

"They were at each other's throats 18 hours a day," said Billy's dad.

His parents were called to the school at least once a week. And worst of all, according to his dad, Billy refused to listen to his parents - ever.

No matter what he did wrong, his mom or dad would talk "until they were blue in the face" and Billy would sit there, fidgeting, with a look on his face that told his parents, "I'm not hearing you. I don't care."

Back when Billy was 5, the teachers suggested to his parents that something was wrong. His parents, John and Laura, took him to a doctor who diagnosed Billy as being hyperactive.

For about 30 days, he was put on medication for the disorder. But because of the controversy then surrounding the use of medication on children, he was taken off the medicine and kept off for the next eight years.

He continued having problems. Billy would try to tell his parents about his day at school - talking a blue streak - and forget what he was saying halfway through the story.

He would try to do his homework and either lose interest in five minutes or discover he didn't bring home the right book, notes, or instructions. Although he was in resource classes at school, he had to struggle to complete homework, study or take tests. Billy often disrupted his classes with sudden outbursts.

His mom said she noticed that Billy would make friends, but would end up fighting with them and scaring them off in a couple of weeks. He ended up hanging around with the crowd of troublemakers at school.

Billy's sister didn't even want to claim him as her brother.

During these years, his parents searched desperately for someone who could help their son. They had always trusted doctors, but no doctor seemed to know what to do for Billy.

Instead of treating him, doctors said he'd grow out of it. Counselors at school offered the family a system of behavior modification using rewards and punishment, but the strict time schedule made Billy even more restless and impulsive.

Teachers and others tried to blame the parents for raising him wrong or not trying hard enough to control him.

Despite everyone's efforts, Billy was still having problems fitting in with people, paying attention in class and getting along at home.

"I never wanted to study. I wanted to be outside or watching TV," Billy said. "In class, it was like I didn't even know what I was saying. Things would just come out."

Laura said they finally reached a point where they wanted to give up. She said they could just look at Billy and tell he was frustrated, too.

That's when they heard about a problem called Attention Deficit Disorder or ADD.

"Billy didn't give us a struggle at all," John said. "It was like he wanted help."

John and Laura took Billy to see a licensed professional counselor.

"When we went in and filled out a questionnaire, every question about ADD fit Billy perfectly," Laura said. Billy's parents were relieved
that someone had finally given a name to a problem
they had lived with for so many years.

But Billy's family was ready for a hopeful
answer after their desperate search. Billy began
taking medication and his mom said they saw
immediate results - a rare occurence, especially
since he was over the age of 12.

"He would come home from school so calm,"
Laura said, "We are living in a different world
now. At first we kept thinking that it was so
nice it couldn't last."

Unfortunately, even after Billy began to improve, his parents had difficulty convincing the
school he had changed.

Billy's parents went though a difficult process
involving loads of paper work and several meetings
before they were able to convince the school
that their son - who had been failing classes in
the spring - would be ready to re-enter the resource program and catch up with his studies.

"We gladly proved every point with them,"
John said. "They didn't want to believe me."

But it is true. Billy's dad said, "Now he actually does what he's told. He'll take up something
for himself - like studying or mowing the yard
- and finish it."

The most rewarding words come from Billy
himself. "Now I'd rather go to the library than
eat lunch."

Billy's friends have changed, and Laura said the change is for the better. He now makes friends and keeps them. "My old friends started telling me, 'You don't do enough,' " Billy said, meaning he didn't cause enough problems to hang around with the trouble makers anymore.

"I feel a lot better about myself," Billy said. "There were people I wanted to know before but couldn't and now I know them."

"It's a joy to have kids like this," Laura said. Our kids are actually friends for the first time."

Now Billy keeps his locker and room neat, he uses dividers to organize his notebooks and he remembers which books to bring home each day. He can even sit still and listen for an hour or more at a time.

Best of all he has long-term goals for his life.

"Before I didn't want to be anything," Billy said. "Now I want to fly, be a pilot - that's all I want to do. That's why I do my math so good."

CASE REPORT

JIM

Jim was referred to me at age 5 for temper outbursts and non-compliant behavior. He was adopted as an infant and his parents reported that he had numerous ear infections, and other childhood illnesses. They reported having difficulty with him at around age 3. He was an only child and the parents had no experience in raising other children.

The initial approach to therapy involved positive and negative reinforcement. Jim would be rewarded for positive behaviors while allowing most negative behaviors to be ignored. This procedure worked occasionally and did succeed in reducing some of his negative behaviors. Counseling with both the parents and Jim continued for a couple of years with limited success. During this time, my familiarity with ADD was growing. I eventually diagnosed him as having ADD and placed him on medication. His behavior improved almost immediately. He still exhibited behavior problems as before but they seemed to be less severe. During these times the behaviors noted were: lying, leaving the house without permission, not finishing chores and talking back to the parents. He was placed in a resource room at school and did fairly well. The parents were extremely co-operative. They spent time with him on homework as well as the extra time needed to explain the reasons for his punishment. At one point the chip reward system was used until it became ineffective. After a few weeks or months it was used again and seemed to be effective. The parents discovered that one system used every day eventually became

boring to Jim. Punishment consisted of brief a-
mounts of time and time out or picking up debris
in the yard. A half gallon milk carton was used
as the measurement. For every misbehavior he
was told he would have to pick up a certain number
of milk cartons of debris.

When attending school meetings, the parents
were questioned as to whether or not they were
expecting too much of the child. In other words
they were blaming the parents for the child's
behavior. The school personnel noted that both
Mr. & Mrs. X were successful and they wondered
if perhaps they were not pushing their adopted
son too hard. Again the school personnel was
looking at the parents as the cause of the child's
behavior, not ADD. When Jim entered puberty,
the medication he was taking had to be changed.
At this point it appeared that the symptoms of
his earlier youth were more pronounced. The medication seemed not to be as effective and his
temper outbursts became more persistent. In other
words, he was getting big enough to think about
physically challenging his parents. The parents
are presently in the process of looking for a placement in a residential facility due to his periodic
temper outbursts.

ATTENTION DEFICIT DISORDERS IN
TWO YOUNG ADULTS

Henry Amado, M.D. AND Patrick J. Lustman, Ph.D.
Washington University, Missouri

Reprinted with Permission of Authors

From Journal of Psychiatric Treatment
And Evaluation, 1983

CASE

Justin P. initially presented to the outpatient psychiatric services of Barnes Hospital in St. Louis in 1976 as a 26-year-old, right-handed, divorced, unemployed, white male with a history of temper outbursts, irritability, poor memory and short attention span, and inability to hold employment for longer than several weeks at a time. He mentioned developing much anxiety in social settings, related to chronic concerns about people allegedly "picking on" him, and often resulting in multiple fights and withdrawal from social activities. Periodically, he would report low mood and despondency, believing himself to be "getting nowhere in life."

The patient had reportedly been a healthy infant, the product of an unremarkable pregancy absent of neonatal complications. He depicted himself as a poor academic student, leaving school in the tenth grade. Parents and teachers did not identify him as having very early sociopathic traits or the classically described hyperkinetic syndrome.

Adolescence and young adulthood constituted chaotic times for the patient. During a two-year

Navy stint, he was involved in frequent fighting, although his discharge was honorable, impulsive acts were common. He sustained a skull fracture and concussion in a motorcycle mishap, with no epileptic sequelae but complaints of severe headaches and memory impairment. He married and divorced three times, conceiving three children. Casual extramarital sex was reported as well. He experimented widely with illicit drugs, including opiates, hallucinogens, barbiturates, and psychostimulants, and engaged in ethanol abuse, typically drinking to excess three nights per week. He attended school sporadically, never obtaining a degree. As mentioned, he was unable to hold steady employment, reportedly becoming too "nervous" and "keyed-up" in the presence of coworkers. When first seen in the outpatient clinic, he was living by himself and described as "rather isolated."

Previously the patient had been admitted to a Veteran's Administration facility on three occasions for violent, destructive behavior (e.g., threatening his father with bodily harm). Diagnoses rendered had included "borderline" personality and drug dependence. An abnormal (but unspecified) EEG was reported during one of the hospitalizations. No consistent follow-up or sustained treatment was forthcoming during this period.

Initial psychiatric assessment at Barnes yielded a complicated and enigmatic picture. The patient at times seemed to describe ideas of reference (e.g., "watching out for what people say under their breath"), passivity experiences (e.g., "feeling physical vibrations from women"), and pseudo-hallucinations (e.g., an externally perceived voice, characterized by the patient as his "subconscious," which would tell him what to do), but there was no clear-cut delusional material, despite persistent probing. He claimed to believe in psychic phenomena, and to have had several "ESP" experiences, which again lacked definite psychotic flavor. Mental status examination was said to be remarkable for jerky, halting delivery of speech, without push or flight of ideas. Informal cognitive testing showed that Justin was disoriented to exact date of the month, could not name the President, and was able to list only three of five major cities requested.

Justin at first received a diagnosis of "undiagnosed psychiatric illness," a term that, while acknowledging the presence of obvious psychiatric disturbance, avoids the pitfalls of premature diagnosis in the face of inadequate information. Differential diagnoses were thought to include such entities as sociopathy, early schizophrenia, "head trauma syndrome," and "explosive personality."

The turning point in this case appears to have come from the patient's own observation that he had noted a calming effect of psychostimulants in the past. An entry in the chart reads:

> The patient watched a TV program on hyperactivity and noted that all symptoms seemed to fit him. He noticed that the treatment was psychostimulants, and remembered how good he felt when he was on speed. Therefore, he presented (today) convinced that he was hyperactive and that Ritalin was the treatment of choice.

As a teenager, the patient had noted that illicit psychostimulants would "make (him) a whole person" because they seemed to have an anxiolytic effect. In those days, he had taken oral agents only, had not experienced euphoriant or paranoid effects, had not become habituated, and had never felt the need to progress to intravenous methods of administration.

A subsequent review of the literature was supportive of the patient's self-diagnosis. Psychological battery was performed and demonstrated left hemisphere dysfunction (on the basis of the Halsted-Reitan), normal intelligence with great variability on verbal subscales of the WAIS, poor memory span and fund of information. Neurological examination was non-focal. CT scan was normal. Nasopharyngeal EEG was declined by the patient.

After an unsuccessful trial of neuroleptic pharmacotherapy, Justin was begun on a cautious regime of methylphenidate, with close monitoring for therapeutic effects, adverse symptoms, and any evidence of medication abuse. There was subsequently gradual but dramatic subjective and objective documentation of improved functioning.

On methylphenidate, the patient appeared less anxious. His thinking had improved in terms of better memory and attention span, although unfortunately a planned repeat psychometric battery was cancelled due to cost. Fighting and antisocial behavior seemed to give way to more productive interactions with others. For the first time in years, he was able to hold part-time, then full-time work in a family-owned construction concern. Psychotic-like, "magical" thinking decreased, as did the halting speech pattern. He enrolled in a Vocational Rehabilitation program. Ethanol, illicit drugs, and sexual promiscuity were all abandoned. In time, he dated steadily and engaged to marry, postponing a formal commitment pending financial security. On the debit side, he had come to ascribe the positive changes in his life as due entirely to the medication, rather than to self-effort as well.

Occasional attempts to decrease the methylphenidate were not successful. Justin would become irritable, sleep poorly, and generally "just feel lousy."

As to this writing, Justin has been stable for four years. The dose of methylphenidate* has been gradually increased to 80mg daily, with adjusting the dose at times so that less is required on non-stressful weekends. He has experienced no side-effects of anorexia, insomnia, weight loss, tachycardia, or jitteriness on the medication. He has shown a remarkable absence of manipulative behavior with regards to procuring medication, and has been a compliant, reliable, and appreciative patient.

*Note that Ritalin was used for this adult. Tofranil has now been found to be the medication of choice for adults.

CASE

Neal S. was first referred for outpatient psychiatric care at Barnes Hospital in the fall of 1978. At the time he was a 23-year-old, right-handed, single, unemployed white male. He had been depressed for three months, developing suicidal ideation which culminated in a serious attempt at overdose with tricyclic medication prescribed by a family physician. After recovering in intensive care, the patient had spent several days in a state mental facility for observation, and had then been referred for outpatient care.

As part of his affective syndrome, Neal described prominent feelings of ennui, which would lead him to renounce jobs and in fact interfered with just about any task requiring persistence. In addition, he described an "inner restlessness," not necessarily accompanied by motoric hyperactivity. Both these problems had been present intermittently for years. He would feel "hyper and irritable," and as though he "had to keep moving all the time." He would also find it difficult to concentrate. Tricyclics had apparently aggravated these "spaced out feelings."

The patient had a history of head injury with unknown sequelae in childhood; he recalled being worked up for a possible seizure disorder in his early teens. He was also hospitalized with encephalitis at age 14. But serial EEG's over the years had all been reported as normal. He had been suspended once, been truant on one occasion, and taken amphetamines one time, with the surprising result of having gone to sleep. From the age of 16 he drank ethanol heavily, almost on a daily basis, in an attempt to self-medicate his depressed mood. He spontaneously stopped drinking at age 20, having escaped the social and physical sequelae of ethanol abuse.

Following a case conference in late 1978, the diagnosis of MBD was advanced, and treatment with psychostimulants was recommended. Due to financial straits, however, the patient stopped attending the clinic for several months, and hence treatment was not implemented until the following spring. He is also attending night school working toward an engineering degree, having the concentration to take difficult mathematical courses. He is active in sports. For financial reasons, he continues to reside with his mother and leads a rather limited social schedule, but is not unhappy with this arrangement. The dosage of methylphenidate has gradually been titrated to 30mg daily in divided doses. There has been no evidence of medication abuse or manipulative behavior toward securing additional supply.

DISCUSSION

These cases illustrate several divergent presentations of ADD in adults. None of the two patients had been specifically identified as having this syndrome as children, but all seemed to have had chronic psychiatric morbidity traceable to their early years. The signs and symptoms previously cited as characteristic of such individuals in the literature are shared to varying extents by the cases here reported. As often seems to occur in psychiatry, it appeared that in each instance a global assessment of the history and clinical presentation may have yielded an accurate diagnosis. Apart from reports of surprising or "paradoxical" responses to casual use of psychostimulants, and the repeated suggestions of nonspecific CNS insult, there did not seem to be definite, unequivocal, or pathognomonic clues to suspect the diagnosis. But in each case, initial lack of familiarity with this diagnostic entity may have resulted in inappropriate pharmacotherapy and delays in implementation of specific treatment. It would stand to reason that the clinician alert to the possibility of ADD persisting in adulthood would be better able to provide optimal care to such patients.

CASE REPORT

JOHN

The following is an excerpt from an interview that a client of mine had with a local newspaper. I would first like to give you some background information. John first heard of me after a relative of his had an appointment. This relative brought their child and I diagnosed him as having ADD. Consequently, the child was placed on medication and improvement was seen in several areas. John witnessed this improvement and also recognized that he seemed to have similar problems when he was a youngster. He felt that he may have had ADD but was never diagnosed.

At our first meeting he was open and honest with his feelings. He related that he had been to several alcohol abuse programs and had been to several psychologists and counselors. The results from these sessions did little to improve his situation. At this point in his life he was rather skeptical of psychologists or anyone connected with the mental health profession. He felt that the same information was repeated at each encounter with a mental health professional. He had spent a large amount of money and started to feel that this was one of the primary motives of most persons in the mental health profession.

Needless to say, he was somewhat skeptical of my ability to help him. Because of his personally witnessing the positive change in his relative, he was willing to see if I could help. After gathering a background and social history I did diagnose him as having ADD. Ironically, at one point in his life he had been placed on the medication normally used for ADD. Unfortunately, he was also placed on another medication. It appeared that the interaction of these two drugs prevented his disorder from being treated properly.

from THE FOCUS
by Curtis Schmidt

ADD VICTIM TALKS OF PAIN, SURVIVAL

Even when he was as young as six or seven, John (not his real name) knew there was something different about him. He was having problems that were not common to his peers.

"I couldn't keep my mind on any one thing for very long. I would fly off the handle real easy and had trouble relating," he comments.

His problems grew progressively worse to the point where he now states "I knew my life was going down the drain all along, but there was no way to stop it, because nobody knew what was wrong."

The "rocky part" of John's life began to surface when he reached his teenage years. "I knew there was something wrong when I was a kid, but I was always real active and could let out my steam in sports," he says. "But when I got to be 13 or 14, things got real bad. My grades declined, I was always getting into fights, and even had a few scrapes with the police."

His parents didn't know what to do and John notes "It was a 'hand up' situation. We all knew something was wrong, but nobody could pin down the source."

So John was sent to the state mental hospital in Big Spring. After little improvement, he moved to Tulsa to live with relatives and re-start high school in a different environment.

That didn't work either as he had more of the same problems and ended up in another mental hospital. He eventually dropped out of high school and moved back to Abilene.

"It was just terrible," he says. "I couldn't concentrate. It was tremendously hard for me to even sit in one place for more than 15 minutes. My temper was worse than ever."

Impulsive as ever, he entered the military service at age 17. "I lied about being in the mental hospitals," he relates.

John went to Vietnam as a rifleman in the infantry. There he began drinking alcoholic beverages on a regular basis and his situation went from bad to worse.

After his tour of duty, he returned home to Abilene and was married after a short relationship. "Another impulsive decision," John says.

Amazingly, the marriage lasted eight years. However, John comments "It was pretty rocky all the time. We were just two people hanging on to each other."

John returned to the service after his divorce. His drinking "continued and got worse" and he became involved with illegal drugs. His temper also grew progressively worse.

After another tour of duty, he returned home again in 1980 and his recreational use of drugs turned into "a daily event," to go along with his drinking problem.

He finally turned to Alcoholics Anonymous in 1983. He "sobered up" and re-married. Things were looking better.

But it didn't last. He gradually fell back into the drinking and drug abuse mode of life. "I was trying to solve the result of the underlying problem but the underlying problem itself remained and just continued to get worse," he says. "I can't believe I survived during all that."

But John did survive and fought back harder than ever. At the age of 31, he sobered up again and started working to attain a college degree, but it wasn't easy. "I really had trouble studying. I mean I had to literally force myself to stick my head inside a book," He says.

Finally, through some friends at college, he learned about ADD (Attention Deficit Disorder) and went to see a local psychotherapist. "He said I fit the bill for ADD perfectly and started me on anti-depressants," John says. The change was "like night and day," he says. "As soon as I started taking the anti-depressants, I found I was able to sit calmly in one place. I could focus my attention on one subject. I wasn't afraid anymore."

John is still working on his comeback, but the improvements are dramatic. His grade point average in college has risen from 1.75 to 2.50 and he is now averaging "B's" in most courses. He has learned to relax and now is looking positively at his future.

He does wonder how his life might have been different if his ailment had been diagnosed earlier, but he is not bitter....just relieved.

"I was dying inside all the time. It could have killed me and almost did," he says. "Sure I wonder how much pain could have been saved if this had been caught when I was five or six, but I really don't have time to worry about that. I've got my life back and a lot of catching up to do."

CASE REPORT

BETTY

The following is a letter from a parent whose daughter was treated for ADD. Before she came for treatment, her grades were poor in comparison to the amount of time she had to put in studying.

If you read between the lines, I believe you will be able to understand the effect that treatment has had on her and those around her.

Dear Glenn,

I just wanted to update you on Betty's progress and to tell you how grateful we are to you for the help you've given her. I'm sending a copy of her report card. The first Six Weeks was before she started treatment, the second Six Weeks started about the same time as the treatment. The first Six Weeks grades still don't show the struggle she has gone through as her grades have always been mostly 60's, 70's, 80's and that's doing below average work and in Tutorial twice a week. Now she's in the Middle and High groups, and isn't in Tutorial since she brought her Reading grade up above 70. We hope she will continue to bring her Reading up some more. But she is just doing so much better. Her teacher said she can see a big difference in her ability to concentrate, finish her work, and she doesn't get so frustrated. At home she is a different child. She's so much calmer, a joy to have as a daughter. Her brothers have changed their attitude with her, treat her like a 10-year old little lady, and enjoy teasing her because she enjoy's being teased. She cooperates when she's told to do something and does some things on her own without being told. She's happy and more mature acting. She and I are rebuilding the relationship we've lost from years of butting heads from morning until night.

I am so thankful to you for what you've done for Betty and all her family. I hope your research and work toward getting this more acknowleged among doctors, teachers, and parents will bring you success. I talked to my doctor here about it and he said he would gladly keep a check on Betty and continue her on Cylert. I told him how pleased we were of her progress.

I also talked to our Superintendent and he's very interested and wants to check into it further.

I wish you would let me know if and when your book comes out and where I can get one. I want to keep up with everything that pertains to ADD. It's so great to know what was causing Betty so much anguish and to be able to help her. The poor child has suffered and gone through so much pain. I could see it in her face everyday. I'm not exaggerating - she now has the most pleasant look of peace of mind on her face. Her self-esteem is coming back and she shares her feelings with me. She's happy - what more can I say, except, everyday I thank God for you and the answer to a prayer.

Sincerely,

Betty's Parents

FINAL COMMENT

The treatment of ADD children at an early age can have a definite impact on our society. I do not feel that I am overstating my position, especially when you consider the research findings mentioned earlier.

Thousands of young people are being mistreated due to the lack of knowledge by the professional community. The biggest offenders are the psychologists, counselors, and others who are not tuned in to the connection between physical and emotional problems.

Aside from ruining the lives of these individuals, millions of tax dollars are being wasted. Again, lack of knowledge is the key factor.

I hope that the individuals reading this book will challenge the knowledge of the professional community by bringing out facts of which few professionals are aware. This may initiate a deeper interest on their part.

If you retain most of the information in this book, I guarantee that you will know more about ADD than most of the professional community.

In the future, I will release another book on ADD. My purpose is not simply to write a book, my purpose is to make our society more aware of ADD.

I hope that through this medium, more people become interested in ADD and this will result in more children being referred for the proper treatment. To accomplish this, it will require you, the reader, to become more involved.

REFERENCES

Alberts-Corush, Jody; Firestone, Phillip, Goodman, John T. Attention and Impulsivity Characteristics of the Biological and Adoptive Parents of Hyperactive and Normal Control Children. American Journal of Orthopsychiatry. Vol. 56 (3). Page 413-423. July 1986.

American Psychiatric Association. DSM III - R, Washington D.C. 1987.

Ayllon, T., & Roberts, M. Eliminating Discipline Problems By Strengthening Academic Performance. Journal of Applied Behavior Analysis, 1974, 7, 71-76.

Ayllon, T., & Rosenbaum, M.S. The Behavioral Treatment of Disruption and Hyperactivity in School Settings. In B. Lahey & A. Kazdin (Eds.), Advances in Child Clincal Psychology (Vol. 1). New York: Plenum, 1977.

Barkley, R. A., & Cunningham, C. E. Do Stimulant Drugs Improve the Academic Performance of Hyperactive Children? Clinical Pediatrics, 1978, 17, 85-92.

Barkley, R.A., & Cunningham, C.E. The Parent-Child Interactions of Hyperactive Children and Their Modification by Stimulant Drugs. In R. Knights & D. Bakker (Eds.), Treatment of Hyperactive and Learning Disordered Children. Baltimore: University Park Press, 1980.

Barkley, R.A., Hyperactive Children. New York: Guilford Press, 1981.

Barkley, R. A., & Ullman, D. A Comparison of Objective Measures of Activity Level and Distractibility in Hyperactive and Nonhyperactive Children. Journal of Abnormal Child Psychology, 1975, 3, 213-224.

Barkley, R. A. A review of stimulant drug research with hyperactive children. Journal of Child Psychology and Psychiatry, 1977, 18, 137-165.

Bassuk, Ellen L. The practitioners guide to psychoactive drugs. 2nd Ed. New York: Plenum Medical Book Co., 1983.

Bell, R. Q. Socialization findings re-examined. In R. Q. Bell & L. Harper (Eds.), Child effects on adults. New York: Wiley, 1977.

168

Bloomingdale, Lewis B. Whither A.D.D. Psychiatric Journal of the University of Ottawa. Vol 9 (4) Dec. 1984.

Brown D., Winsberg B., Bialer I., et al: Imipramine therapy and seizures. Three children treated for hyperactive behavior disorders. Am J Psychiatry 130: 210–212, 1972.

Bryant, Ernest T., Scott, Monte L., Golden, Charles J., Tori, Christopher D. Nueropsychological Deficits, Learning Disability, and Violent Behavior. Vol. 52 (2) 323–324, 1984.

Campbell, S. Mother-child interaction in reflective, impulsive, and hyperactive children. Developmental Psychology, 1973, 8, 341–347.

Cantwell, D. P. Psychiatric illness in the families of hyperactive children. Archives of General Psychiatry, 1972, 27, 414–427.

Cantwell, D. P., & Satterfield, J. H. The prevalence of academic underachievement in hyperactive children. Journal of Pediatric Psychology, 1978, 3, 168–171.

Cantwell, D. P. A clinician's guide to the use of stimulant medication for the psychiatric disorders of children. Developmental and Behavioral Pediatrics, 1980, 1, 133–140.

Cantwell, D. P., & Carlson, G. A. Stimulants. In J. Werry (Ed.), Pediatric psychopharmacology. New York: Brunner/Mazel, 1978.

Cantwell, Dennis P. The Attention Deficit Disorder Syndrome, Current Knowledge, Future needs. Journal of the American Academy of Child Psychiatry. Vol. 23 (3), 315–318, May 1984.

Caparulo, Barbara K., Cohen, Donald J., Rothman, Stephen L., Young, Gerald J., Katz, Jonathan D., Shaywitz, Sally E., Shaywitz, Bennett A. Computed Tomographic Brain Scanning in Children with Developmental Neuropsychiatric Disorders. Annual progress in child psychiatry and child development. New York, Brunner/Mazel, 1982.

Clampit, M. K., Pickle, Jane B. Stimulant medication and the hyperactive Adolescent: Myths and Facts. Adolescence, Vol. 18, (72), 812–822, Winter 1983.

Cohen, Arie; Lufi Dubi. Using the WISC-R to identify Attentional Deficit Disorder. Psychology in Schools. Vol. 22 (1), 40–42. Jan. 1985.

Conners, C. K., & Taylor, E. Pemoline, Methylphenidate, and placebo in children with minimal brain dysfunction. Archives of General Psychiatry, 1980, 37, 922-932.

Conners, C. K. Food additives and hyperactive children. New York: Plenum, 1980.

Douglas, V. I., & Peters, K. G. Toward a clearer definition of the attentional deficit of hyperactive children. In G. A. Hale & M. Lewis (Eds.), Attention and the development of cognitive skills. New York: Plenum, 1980.

Feingold, B. Why your child is hyperactive. New York: Random House, 1975.

Fleisher, Lisa S., Soodak, Leslie C., Jelin, Marjorie A. Selective Attention Deficits in Learning Disabled Children: Analysis of the Data Base. Exceptional children, Vol. 51, No. 2, 136-141, Oct. 1984.

Gaddes, W. H. Learning disabilities and brain function: A neuropsychological approach. New York: Springer-Verlag, 1980.

Gillberg, Carina I; Gillberg, Christopher. Three Year Follow-up at age 10 of children with minor neurodevelopmental Disorders I: Behavioural Problems. Developmental medicine and child neurology. Vol. 25 (4), 438-449, Aug. 1983.

Golden, C. J., Hammeke, T. A., & Purisch, A. D. The Luria-Nebraska neuropsychological battery. Los Angeles: Western Psychological Services, 1980.

Goyete, C. H., Conners, C. K., & Ulrich, R. F. Normative data on revised Conners parent and teacher rating scales. Journal of Abnormal Child Psychology, 1978, 6, 221-236.

Harley, J. P., Ray, R. S., Tomasi, L., Eichman, P. L., Matthews, C. G., Chun, R., Cleeland, C. S., & Traisman, E. Hyperkinesis and food additives: Testing the Feingold hypothesis. Pediatrics, 1978, 61, 818-828.

Harley, J. P., Matthews, C. G., & Eichman, P. L. Synthetic food colors and hyperactivity in children: A double-blind challenge experiment. Pediatrics, 1978, 62, 975-983.

Hecaen, H., & Albert, M. L. Human neuropsychology. New York: Wiley, 1978.

Heliman, K. M., & Valenstein, E. Clinical neuropsychology. New York: Oxford University Press, 1979.

Horn, Wade F.; Chatoor, Irene; Conners, Keith C. Addictive Effects of Dexedrine and Self-Control Training. Behavior Modification. Vol. 7 (3), 383-402, 1983.

Humphries, T., Kinsbourne, M., & Swanson, J. Stimulant effects on cooperation and social interaction between hyperactive children and their mothers. Journal of Child Psychology and Psychiatry, 1978, 19, 13-22.

Hussey, Hans R., Howell, David C. Relationships Between Adult Alcoholism and Childhood Behavior Disorders. Psychiatric Journal of the University of Ottawa. Vol. 10, (2), 114-119, June 1985.

Kendall, P. C., & Wilcox, L. E. Self-control in children: Development of a rating scale. Journal of Consulting and Clincial Psychology, 1979, 47, 1020-1029.

Kinsbourne, M., & Caplan, P. J. Children's learning and attention problems. Boston: Little, Brown, 1979.

Lahey, B. B. Behavior therapy with hyperactive and learning disabled children. New York: Oxford University Press, 1979.

Linnoila M., Gualtieri T., Jobson K., et al: Characteristics of the therapeutic response to imipramine in hyperactive children. Am J Psychiatry 136: 1201-1203, 1979.

Mash, E. J., & Dalby, J. T. Behavioral interventions for hyperactivity. In R. Trites (Ed.), Hyperactivity in children: Etiology, measurement, and treatment implications. Baltimore: University Park Press, 1979.

Mash, E. J., & Terdal, L. G. (Eds.). Behavioral assessment of childhood disorders. New York: Guilford, 1981.

Molitch, M., & Eccles, A. K. Effects of benzedrine sulphate on intelligence scores of children. American Journal of Psychiatry, 1937, 94, 587-590.

Morganstern, K. P. Behavioral interviewing: The initial stages of assessment. A practical handbook. New York: Pergamon, 1976.

Morrison, J. R., & Stewart, M. A. A family study of the hyperactive child syndrome. Biological Psychiatry, 1971, 3, 189-195.

Morrison, J. R., & Stewart, M. A. The psychiatric status of the legal families of adopted hyperactive children. Archives of General Psychiatry, 1973, 28, 888-891.

Ownby, Raymond L. The Neuropsychology of Attention Deficit Disorders in Children. Journal of Psychiatric Treatment and Evaluation. Vol 5, 229-236, 1983.

Patterson, G. R. The aggressive child: Victim and architect of a coercive system. In E. J. Mash, L. A. Hamerlynck, & L. C. Handy (Eds.), Behavior modification and families. New York: Brunner/Mazel, 1976.

Pattison, Mansell. Clinical Approaches to the Alcoholic Patient. Psychosomatics, Vol. 27, (11), 762-770, Nov. 1986.

Psyche-Media Inc. The Hyperactive client. Psychiatric Aspects of Mental Retardation Reviews, Vol. 3 (3), March 1984.

Rapoport, Judith L. Antidepressants in childhood Attention Deficit Disorder and Obsessive Compulsive Disorder. Psychosomatics. Vol. 27 (11), Nov. 1986.

Reid, William H. Treatment of the DSM III psychiatric disorders. New York: Brunner/Mazel, 1983.

Roche, A. F., Lipman, R. S., Overall, J. E., & Hung, W. The effects of stimulant medication on the growth of hyperkinetic children. Pediatrics, 1979, 63,847-850.

Safer, R. P., & Allen, D. J. Hyperactive children: Diagnosis and management. Baltimore: University Park Press, 1976.

Sleator, E. K., & Ullman, R. K. Can the physician diagnose hyperactivity in the office? Pediatrics, 1981, 67, 13-17.

Smith, L. Your child's behavior chemistry. New York: Random House, 1975.

Solomons, G. Drug therapy: Initiation and follow-up. Annals of the New York Academy of Science, 1973, 205, 335-344.

Sprague, R., & Sleator, E. Methylphenidate in hyperkinetic children: Differences in dose effects on learning and social behavior. Science, 1977, 198,1274-1276.

Stare, F. J., Whelan, E. M., & Sheridan, M. Diet and hyperactivity: Is there a relationship? Pediatrics, 1980, 66, 521-525.

Swanson, J., & Kinsbourne, M. Food dyes impair performance of hyperactive children on a laboratory learning test. Science, 1980, 207, 1485-1486.

Taylor, E. Food additives, allergy, and hyperkinesis. Journal of Child Psychology and Psychiatry, 1979, 20, 357-363.

Varley, Christopher K. Diet and the Behavior of children with Attention Deficit Disorder. Journal of the American Academy of Child Psychiatry, 23, 2: 182-185,1984.

Waizer I., Hoffman S., Polizos P., et al: Outpatient treatment of hyperactive school children with imipramine. Am J Psychiatry 131: 587-591, 1975.

Weiss, B., Williams, J. H., Margen, S., Abrams, B., Caan, B, Citron, L., Cox, C., McKibben, J., Ogar, D., & Schultz, S. Behavioral responses to artificial food colors. Science 1980, 207, 1487-1488.

Wender, E. Food additives and hyperkinesis. American Journal of Diseases of Children, 1977, 131, 1204-1206.

Wender, P. H. Minimal brain dyfunction in children. New York: Wiley, 1971.

Williams, J. I., Cram, D. M., Tausig, F. T., & Webster, E. Relative effects of drugs and diet on hyperactive behaviors: An experimental study. Pediatrics, 1978, 61, 811-817.

Winsbery B. G.: Effects of imipramine and dextroamphetamine on behavior of neuropsychiatrically impaired children. Am J Psychiatry 128: 1425-1431.

ORDER FORM

To get other copies of this book, you can order them through your local bookstore or directly from:

> Forresst Publishing
> (Glenn Hunsucker)
> P.O. Box 7046
> Abilene, Texas 79608

Please send _____ copies of ATTENTION DEFICIT DISORDER at $12.95 per copy, plus shipping charges of $2.00 for the first book and 50¢ for each additional book to:

Name:_____

Address:_____

City: _____

State: _____ Zip: _____

Phone: (_____)_____

If you are interested in subscribing to a quarterly newsletter on ADD, please contact Forresst Publishing for the details.

ABOUT THE AUTHOR

Glenn Hunsucker has a private practice in counseling in Abilene, Texas. He received his Bachelor's Degree from Hardin Simmons University and his Master's Degree in Psychology from Abilene Christian University. He is licensed by the State of Texas as a Professional Counselor and has a variety of professional experience. He has taught psychology at the collegiate level as well as conducted lectures around the country. He has done management counsulting and has authored a weekly newspaper column.

He has been Administrator of a child care facility for difficult teens and has done extensive work with families and children. He consults with Juvenile Probation Departments, Department of Human Services, and Public School Systems.

He holds memberships in the Texas Association For Counseling and Development and the American Association for Counseling and Development. He has received numerous honors and awards for his work with children. He was recently nominated for listing in Who's Who Among Human Service Professionals, 1988.

He is currently Director of two ADD Screening Centers in Abilene and Ft. Worth, Texas.